DEEP LIVING

DEEP LIVING

DEEP LIVING

Healing Yourself
To Heal The Planet

Susanne Meyer-Fitzsimmons

FCP

Full Court Press
Englewood Cliffs, New Jersey

First Edition

Copyright © 2016 by Susanne Meyer-Fitzsimmons

Published in the United States of America
by Full Court Press, 601 Palisade Avenue,
Englewood Cliffs, NJ 07632
fullcourtpressnj.com

ISBN 978-1-938812-87-3
Library of Congress Catalog No. 2016958598

Book design by Barry Sheinkopf for Bookshapers.Com
(www.bookshapers.com)

Cover art by Caroline Siecke-Pape

Colophon by Liz Sedlack

To Brian, Nicholas and Zoë,
and of course my parents

DISCLAIMER

Because of the dynamic nature of the internet, any web addresses or links contained in this book may have changed since publication and may no longer be valid.

The views expressed in this book are solely those of the author and do not necessarily reflect the views of the publisher, and the publisher hereby disclaims any responsibility for them.

The author of this book does not dispense medical advice or prescribe the use of any technique as a form of treatment for physical, emotional, or medical problems without the advice of a physician, either directly or indirectly. The intent of the author is only to offer information of a general nature to help you in your quest for emotional and spiritual wellbeing. In the event you use any of the information in this book for yourself, which is your constitutional right, the author and the publisher assume no responsibility for your actions.

ACKNOWLEDGMENTS

No book gets created in a vacuum, and this one has been a lifetime in the making. Accordingly, the list of thank-yous is long. So, sincere general thanks to all the wonderful people who contributed directly or indirectly to its making.

More specifically:

To my parents, who were instrumental in developing my critical-thinking skills and inspired my passion for food, cooking, travel, good conversation, culture, and entertaining.

To my husband Brian, who has had to listen to this book idea for the past seven years and has been so supportive and encouraging in so many ways; to my son Nicholas, who has patiently, and sometimes not so patiently, listened to and participated in many a spirited cultural discussion, and who has developed strong instincts for culturally critical thinking himself; and to my daughter Zoë, who practices every day of her life many of the things I preach.

To my country and its partially horrible history, which sent me on my initial spiritual quest as a teenager. Maybe it has redeemed itself a bit.

To all my graduate professors at ESC, who each helped formulate one aspect of the research that went into the making of this book: Elana Michelson, for shaping my graduate program and, indirectly, the structure of this volume, with much wisdom and insight, and for suggesting I take a course in creative non-fiction writing (bingo!); to Eric Zencey, for making sure I wasn't veering too far off the academic-thinking path during the consciousness evolution research that went into Part Three; to Ruth Silver, for shaping my research on holistic nutrition; to Kelsea Habecker, for introducing me to creative non-fiction writing, book proposals, query letters, and the whole platform business, and as second adviser on my final project, which was my first book draft; to Anastasia Pratt, for guiding my research on the non-violence movement and compassionate communication; to Julie Evans, who witnessed the Quantum Healing course morph from researching alternative healing modalities to defining health and healing in a much, much broader sense (which informs the entire book), for being my first thesis adviser and shaping the raw product for the book, and for commenting on the final book draft; to Kate Forbes, for her research guidance in Integral Agriculture; to Lorraine Lander, for her wise guidance and the great phone conversations we had about the research that went into the Ecology for the Future course; to Sabrina Fuchs-Adams, Susan Hollis, and Nan Travers for honing my research, writing, and critical-thinking skills.

To Larry Dossey and Marcey Shapiro, physicians and authors, who keep expanding how we heal by rewriting the narrative, and for contributing blurbs for this book so willingly and early on in the process; it means a lot to me, thank you.

To Lewis Mehl-Madrona, physician, author, and medical narrator, who so patiently read all my requests for blurbs over the past years and found the time in his busy schedule to send me one; thank you.

To Michele Galante, M.D., homeopathic physician extraordinaire, my medical and consciousness hero.

To my book GC Barry Sheinkopf, who did it all: editing for content, good English (Chicago style!), and my iffy comma skills, for designing the book, and for formatting the eBook, getting it printed, registered, and on to Amazon and B&N.

To Ray and Terry Boswell, who both kept nudging me to contact Barry.

To Caroline Siecke-Pape, who not only designed my original website with its lovely graphics, but also created the book cover.

To Inez Freund and Eileen Patterson of Creative Vision, who helped me establish my platform from early marketing to formulating my website message, setting up my social media accounts, early talks, educating me on palm cards, and being faithful cheerleaders all along.

To my most enthusiastic blog follower, Annette Sanchez, who said long ago, "You don't have to go to church when you read Susanne's blog, it's so spiritual," and who kept asking when the book would be published. Here it is, finally, Annette.

To my writer's group: Jane Bloom and Claudia Myers for listening and commenting on bits and pieces of this work over the past year or so; and chocolate writer and lover Micki Shortess-Smith, for introducing me to David Wolfe and his Superfoods, and bringing the most delicious chocolate treats to our meetings.

To Tom Mattingly and Sharon Linnéa, who told me that the manuscript had some merit, and for their enlightening writers' workshop where I met Jane, Claudia, and Micki, who became my writer's group.

To Bay NVC for their permission to reprint their Universal Human Needs and Feelings/Emotions list.

To Barbara Bash, Imre Berty, and Roberta Wall, from whom I got the Universal Human Needs and Feelings/Emotions list at the Sky Lake Lodge retreat *Speaking True Listening Deep,* and for their indirect contributions to the chapter on communication.

Finally, to Arne Naess, deep ecologist extraordinaire and philospher, who coined the term "Deep Ecology" way back when, and who inspired my title.

Preface

Awakening slowly and gradually from a deep mental slumber to the realization that I am in charge of my life was an empowering insight. The conclusions I have come to over the past few years might be called "deep" or "holistic" living. This book is about defining such a holistic life, a life worth living; a meaningful, joyful and fulfilled life in co-creation and harmony with our planet, Nature, and my fellow men—including you. It is about creating a world you and I can be proud to pass on to our children and grandchildren, and to our great-great-great-great-grandchildren, as Native Americans might say, projecting seven generations out. It is about taking charge and being responsible, personally and as a society, by making choices that are good for you and me individually, good for all our fellow human beings, and good for the planet at large, creating win-win situations across the board.

To me, life is about self-realization through interaction with others and our environment. Living holistically is living with deep awareness and in tune and harmony with ourselves and others, with spirit and our surroundings. The word "holistic" comes from "whole," encompassing the entire spectrum of life, both seen and unseen, physical and spiritual, quantitative and qualitative aspects. Thus, the term *deep living* refers to a balanced and inclusive life with intensity and meaning. Counting the calories of a piece of cheese without considering the yummy factor is unexciting and conveys only half the story.

Currently, we are experiencing a huge paradigm shift in real time. Look at the many natural and man-made disasters, look at our broken environment, look at our politics, look at the sad supermarket foods, look at the many people in distress. Things are messy; things are in turmoil. The old order is being undone, and a new order is breaking through from underneath. It's scary and exciting. It's scary if you live through it without vision and understanding of what's going on and let yourself passively be carried by the stream of events. It's exciting if you are aware of what's happening and consciously participate in the renewal process by playing an active and creative part in it. But in order to participate, you need to have a vision. In this book, I am suggesting possible holistic visions for five everyday aspects of life that are cooperative, compassionate, sustainable, and meaningful.

- Nature, our relationship with it, how to care for and relate to our environment thoughtfully
- Agriculture, our relationship with it, how to grow food in the most healthful, beneficial, and sustainable ways
- Food, our relationship with it, and how to nourish ourselves in the most wholesome way
- People, our relationships, and how to relate to one another compassionately
- Body, our relationship with it, how to care for our body, soul, and spirit through an integral understanding of the human being

Let's visualize together how to interact with nature in co-operative and co-creative ways; how to grow food so it is wholesome, densely packed with nutrients, and contributes to the environment's renewal; how food can benefit and heal in addition to nourishing the soul; how to communicate so people feel embraced and relationships can heal; and how a holistic understanding of the body can gently move us forward on our personal path to fulfillment. This process takes awareness, reflection, initiative, perseverance, work and courage. My examples may serve as illustration or inspiration, but the experiences on your own journey towards self-fulfillment will be different. Your own answers will come from within, from the deeper you. Your answers will be entirely unique to you. They will be your very own solutions to the best possible life you can live. Imagine the liberating freedom, and awesome responsibility!

When you function in harmony with yourself and nature (or spirit, or God, or whatever else you feel comfortable calling it), you feel content, happy, fulfilled, rewarded, elated, appreciative, or creative. When you are disconnected from those elements, it hurts, it grates, you feel unfulfilled, out-of-sorts, irritated, nervous, fearful, anxious, and you may ultimately become physically ill. Many live like that, at war with each other, at war with the environment, at war with their body, at war with spirit and soul, at war with themselves. We see this reflected in what is happening in the world, in how disrespectfully people speak with each other, in how brutally we interact with the environment, in how unaware a fashion we treat our bodies, and in how callously we handle our food supply. As a result it is not surprising that so many people resort to consumerism or anti-depressants in their confused search for a better life, and that so many teenagers retreat into the virtual cyber world or even commit suicide out of sheer desperation. And while this un-ease began as a specifically Western cultural and existential crisis, it is now also taking hold in countries like India and China as they are beginning to embrace a Western lifestyle and its values.

But this book's primary purpose is not about criticizing what is, although comparison and criticism help at first to clarify what we *don't* want. It is about modeling what a holistic, fulfilling life might look like, and to help you create it for yourself. It is about the power of possibilities. After all, life is what you make it, as they say. I did not fully understand what that means until I went through a brief period of depression, during which I saw myself as a victim of life and circumstances. Once that had sunk in, though, I pulled myself up by the boot straps and brought a prescription for an anti-depressant back to the pharmacy, realizing that I was the creator of everything around me, my relationships, my profession, my surroundings, my depression, my dreams and endless possibilities. I shifted my outlook from victim to creator in order to create what I wanted.

We have generally been taught that thinking of oneself is selfish, but that is a misinterpretation. Opting out of being belittled is not selfish. Opting out of being abused is not selfish. It is actually necessary to rid your life of things that are not beneficial for you, so you can be who you need to be in your heart. Only when you are fully the best you can be can you also have an inspiring, strengthening, and positive influence on everyone around you. You must be inspired to be inspiring, and you can only be inspired if you have empowering influences in your life. When you are satisfied with yourself, in tune with who you are— the French call it *être bien dans sa peau*, feeling good inside your skin—then that positivity reverberates all around you, like the ripple effect of a pebble thrown into water. Many people who then come in contact with your life-affirming energy, charisma, and radiance usually send it right back your way through smiles, kind words, and gestures. Becoming healthy is not only good for *you*, it is also beneficial for everyone around you. Healing the world through healing yourself is not a new thought. Here, then, is to that old adage. This book is about healing yourself in order to heal our wounded planet.

—S. M-F.

Warwick, New York

TABLE OF CONTENTS

PART ONE
Life and Healing

Chapter 1: Head and Heart, *1*

Chapter 2: Health Is a Cultural Product, *10*

Chapter 3: How We Heal, And Who Does It, *22*

PART TWO
Reinventing Our Connections

Chapter 4: Man As Part of Nature, Not Apart from Nature, *41*

Chapter 5: Healthy Soil = Healthy Environment = Healthy Body, *66*

Chapter 6: Food to Nourish, Not Food As Fuel, *94*

Chapter 7: Relationships and Communication:
Why Talking Nice Is So Nice, *123*

Chapter 8: The Body, and a New Way to Heal, *142*

PART THREE
The Bigger Picture, and Why All of This Is Really Important

Chapter 9: A Broader Perspective, *171*

Appendix A: *Suggested Further Reading by Chapter Subject*, *183*

Appendix B: *Universal Human Needs*, *188*

Feelings / Emotions, *190*

PART ONE
Life And Healing

"You must be the change you wish to see in the world."
—Mahatma Gandhi (1869–1948)

"One sees clearly only with the heart. What is essential is invisible to the eye."
—Antoine de Saint-Exupéry (1900–1944)
The Little Prince

Chapter 1

HEAD AND HEART

The long-neglected importance of our inner life

LISTENING TO YOUR HEART is often snubbed by our culture. *Emotional* can be a bad word. But where did we end up by ignoring our hearts' messages, by choosing with our "rational" heads instead of our "emotional" hearts? Rational, and with it scientific, thought is generally looked upon as "good," while emotional awareness has often been tagged as "bad" or, well, "irrational." Many of us find emotions and feelings embarrassing, in addition to which we don't quite understand their role and place. What happened to our inner life?

Although information about our unsustainable and destructive ways has been widely available in print for several decades now, it is human nature to resist change, and we have tried to ignore the messages. Yet it is an indisputable fact that we have been environmentally trashing, pillaging, and raping our planet Earth, that same Earth from which everything we need to live comes; that people have become overweight and sick from eating manufactured foods; and that many of our expensive medical procedures are unwarranted, very invasive, and don't necessarily make us any healthier.

Because our culture has become so singularly head- and dollar-oriented, everything in mainstream culture seems to boil down to *how much* and *how fast*, instead of *how well*. Our food purchases hinge on *how much money* and *how many nutrients* instead of *how wholesome and tasty*; our doctor visits revolve around *how much money* and *how quickly*, not *how caring* and *how effective*; and even our ways of communication boil down to *how fast* and *how direct*, instead of *how compassionate* and *how uplifting*. In reaction, there is a definite uneasiness about life in general, although most people cannot put their finger on what exactly is wrong. Many are frustrated or irritated at best, strung out or ill at worst. These days teenagers go through one of the most important phases of life without the meaningful direction of their elders, because many adults, too, are confused or depressed, not knowing where to turn for answers, help, advice, and direction.

It is frustrating to ceaselessly hear in so many ways that our unseen reality, our thoughts, emotions, intuitions, and beliefs, are irrational, or unimportant, or irrelevant, and always to be reminded to be rational (meaning choosing with your head, even if your heart says otherwise). The fuzzy terminology for our unseen reality expresses our general confusion about it. Yet existence clearly consists of both a material and spiritual side, a seen and an unseen aspect, the material and the metaphysical, which is simply not acknowledged in much of mainstream Western culture. We are quite clear on what the material part consists of—everything we can see, feel, hear, taste, and smell with our five senses, because we have learned to measure and manipulate this material reality. We just *know* it is *real*. The spiritual aspect of life, our emotions and feelings, thoughts and beliefs, dreams, values, symbols, and stories, everything that makes up our consciousness, seems more vague and less real—and I will explain why in Chapter 2. Many people don't understand or believe that we can manipulate this aspect or inspect it scientifically. Many more who may be open to such thinking are not quite sure how to do so. Most of the time we sweep that side under the rug, while, for example, Native Americans or Buddhists *embrace* the spiritual and inner component of life. Even the *word* spiritual is suspect in our culture. It is full of mystery, linked to religion, not clearly definable for many. Due to cultural pressure, we often try to hide our emotions. But bottling them up does not help. Former U.S. House of Representatives Speaker John Boehner was relentlessly teased about his teary-eyedness, which occurred every time he connected with his emotional side, his heart and soul. But it's *through* our emotions, beliefs, and thoughts that we express and reveal our inner selves. Our emotions are indicators of how much or how little we are in tune with the world around us. Positive emotions like love, exuberance, pleasure, or joy are a sign of deep affirmative connection. My heart laughs when the sky is a brilliant blue, the sun shines, and my daughter comes jumping and smiling off the school bus. In that moment, everything is perfect. Negative emotions like fear, irritation, nervousness, anger, or despondency indicate dislike or discomfort, and the need to either confront the issue that triggered it or eliminate it from one's life.

With regard to the state of the world, who actually wants environmental damage, or war, or to be stressed and sick? Nobody. So how and why did we get what we don't want? Are we innocent victims? It seems so contradictory that we live in a world that is not at all as we would want it to be if we had our choice. It's as if something had gone awry and created a big mess. Why is that? And what to do? This chapter proposes answers to why we're where we're at as a culture. It also paves the way for Part Two, on how to turn things around and to shape your reality according to your inner truth. It's a matter of really opening your heart and mind, really listening, and taking the incredible responsibility for making changes in your life, even if they may seem cumbersome at first. It is about living life to its fullest, or walking the talk. Don't get me wrong about rational thinking. It absolutely has its purpose, and we'll hear more about it in Part Three. But there needs to be a balance, and we tend to ignore the heart or emotional side much of the time. Here are some fundamental thoughts that lead to a better understanding of how our reality gets shaped and why things are the way they are.

Beliefs, thoughts, and values, and how they shape our personal reality

Like a mirror, life reflects back to you what you put out. Your physical reality shapes itself around values, thoughts, and beliefs you hold. This idea may seem far out, but understanding it is crucial to the rest of the book, and to understanding how life on Earth functions. Let me illustrate how thoughts create reality with the example of the house we just built.

When we moved out of Manhattan as a youngish couple over twenty years ago, the old house we bought then suited our needs. But as we grew up and our lifestyle changed, so did those needs.

We now wanted privacy and quiet (our old house was on the road); a very energy-efficient house (the one we'd been in for so long was over two hundred years old, drafty, and costly to heat); a redefined living environment (our lifestyle had changed so much in all those years); and a little more space (for teenage children, two cats, and two home offices). We realized our wish a few years ago by buying a beautiful private wooded piece of property. Then we came up with a list of space and adjacency requirements, aesthetic desires, mechanical parameters, energy requirements, and, of course, budgetary constraints. After we paid off the property over a number of years, we hired an architect, completed the design, arranged for financing, and hired a contractor—all signs of sufficient creative energy to make it happen. When we moved into our net-zero house two years ago, thoughts had crystallized into matter. If we had wavered along the way, been unable to make up our minds, the house could not have happened, because it would have lacked the creative energy behind it.

The more precisely we were able to define our needs and wishes beforehand, and the better the architect and contractor were able to translate them, the more the finished house would be able to fulfill our needs and reflect our lifestyle. It's now a reflection of who we currently are, of our needs, beliefs, and values. The process shows how an idea moves from the unseen to the seen, how it begins as a thought and manifests in the physical if, and once, there is enough creative energy behind it. All things begin in thought form, but only those with enough energy and momentum behind them materialize.

The work of biologists Humberto Maturana and Francisco Varela clads this process in a scientific theory. Their *Santiago The-*

ory of Cognition says, in short, that consciousness or information makes up one half of our reality, while matter makes up the other. Action is fueled by consciousness and is the propelling creative force that leads from idea (or the spiritual, or the unseen) to matter (or the physical, or the seen). *Every material thing, every manifestation, begins in the mind.*

In fact, let's continue with the house example and take it a step further to inspect how values shape reality. You can read your personal values in your house or apartment. Neighborhood, style and size of house or apartment, types of rooms and their usage, types of furnishings, type of home decor and colors, all say a lot about the homeowner. Businessman David Siegel and his wife Jackie's unfinished ninety-thousand-square-foot would-be château, portrayed in the 2012 documentary *The Queen of Versailles*, says everything about the couple's values. *Your personal life is shaped by your beliefs and values. To change your life you need to change your beliefs and values.*

Your values and beliefs are part of your inner or spiritual self, and manifest around you in the material world. If you don't like what you see in your life, inspect the values and beliefs that created it. Once they are clear to you, you are in a better position to change them.

Beliefs, thoughts, and values—how they shape our cultural reality

Like a mirror, our culture, too, reflects back to us values, thoughts, and beliefs that formed it. When many people have similar beliefs and values, they show up in the culture, which we, and our ancestors, have shaped collectively through our accumulated values and beliefs, and we are observing and living the effects of the beliefs and values that built this culture. Germany unplugged its eight oldest nuclear reactors a few years ago, almost half of all German reactors, in reaction to the Japanese Fukushima nuclear disaster. Although it remains to be seen how practical and realistic this act was, it demonstrated that country's strong environmental concerns and values.

Similarly, American college education today has become very costly. Average tuition has risen exponentially in recent years and is entirely out of proportion with the cost of living. In comparison to other countries, it seems that universities here have relegated our children's education to second place behind the urge for continuous growth and profit. Education has become for-profit, which it shouldn't be, but that is clearly another expression of dominant values. If you don't like what you see culturally, politically, environmentally, vote, become engaged locally, help shape your community. Such involvement can move mountains. Because of just such public pressures, New York State recently banned fracking, and the minimum wage is being raised. It always starts with you and me.

You can take any cultural aspect of this or any other country, and read the values and beliefs that created it. What about the absence of a substantial Green Party in the U.S.? What about the melding of religion and government in Muslim countries? What about Bhutan's Gross National Happiness Index? And how about the tight genetically modified organism (GMO) regulations in many countries (and their absence in this one)? They all reveal each culture's priorities, beliefs, and values.

Culture is created by the collective beliefs and values of a majority of believers. The culture changes when a majority of believers shift their beliefs and values. This can happen either gradually and peacefully, or abruptly through a revolutionary or radical process, depending on when and how critical mass has been reached.

Cultures change from the inside out, that is to say, grassroots-style, from changes in personally held values and beliefs, whose effects accumulate exponentially the more people adopt new values, until they come to a tipping point. By personally changing and healing destructive, aggressive, or unsustainable behavior, you radiate out the new behavior, and with enough momentum from others who do the same, the culture eventually adjusts, shifts, and begins to form new values. The peaceful Occupy Wall Street Movement, and Senator Bernie Sanders' surprising rise and success in the 2016 presidential campaign, are recent manifestations of just such changes in values. Capitalism worked well in this country as long as everyone could believe that the American dream was achievable. However, in recent years our economic system has evolved towards the top one percent possessing most of the power and earning most of the income. The awareness of the ninety-nine percent who have been left increasingly behind has generated enough will and energy that the movement has also spread to cities beyond the U.S. It is now simply called the Occupy Movement, and its premise has spread to other movements such as Occupy Monsanto. "The human community evolves through the evolution of the individual," writes the Teilhard de Chardin scholar Vincent Frank Bedogne.

Throughout this book, I have attempted to dig up the value and belief system behind our present culture and making an argument for the timeliness of rebalancing and healing it. By listening increasingly to our hearts' messages, we can collectively shift to a sustainable, rewarding, cooperative, and deeply meaningful holistic lifestyle. In the following chapter, I will get to what health and healing in the larger sense actually mean, and how that relates to healing our individual lives and our Western culture.

Chapter 2

HEALTH IS A
CULTURAL PRODUCT

Does health mean only that nothing hurts?

HEALTH IS WHEN NOTHING HURTS, RIGHT? Not so fast. Asking what health actually means is one of the most fundamental questions you can ask yourself. We all strive for happiness, nobody wants to suffer, and most of us feel emotional pain when we see others suffer. I am happiest when my husband and my children laugh and enjoy life, and it makes me cry to see pictures of children or animals suffering, children injured by natural disasters, or the victims of man-made calamities like war or environmental damage. We have a natural desire to reestablish a state of health and harmony—to *ourselves*, so *we* can be happy and enjoy life—and also to those who suffer, both so *they* can be happy and enjoy life, but also to avoid watching them suffer. We don't always realize how dependent we are on each others' happiness. Martin Luther King said it perhaps best: "Strangely enough, I can never be what I ought to be until you are what you ought to be. You can never be what you ought to be until I am what I ought to be."

To return to a definition of health, the issue is deeper than merely looking at the physical body because we need to include the mind. Yet much of mainstream culture still subscribes to something like this: "Health is the absence of illness," or "Health is soundness of body."

According to those definitions, from the *Online Oxford Reference* and the *Oxford Universal Dictionary,* respectively, white collar criminal Bernie Madoff might be healthy on the surface. Yet something in criminals is completely out of balance, and it is not the body, it's the mind. Granted, we do acknowledge mental illness. But excessive materialism, for example, is not considered a mental illness or even an imbalance; it is even worshiped in our culture. And many consider mind and body independent from one another, too. If we dig deeper, though, we can find a more complete definition of health, such as the one from a recent dissertation by Anita Chambers entitled "An Emerging Theory of Health as Unified Coherence": "Health is a state of coherence and unity of one's body, mind, and spirit."

You may wonder how various definitions of health can even coexist. The word *health* comes from Old English and means *whole*. Interestingly, it comes from the same root as *holy*. The differing definitions of health reflect two opposing worldviews in the Western world. Much of Western culture has, seemingly, been on a trajectory of descent into the material for the past several hundred years, to the almost complete exclusion, and even denial, of the existence of the spiritual, making science its God instead. But while many keep holding on to a strictly material world image, this picture is starting to fray along the edges. In fact, a growing number of scientists —like cell biologist Bruce Lipton, biologist Rupert Sheldrake, physicians Deepak Chopra and Larry Dossey, or the late UCLA energy healing researcher Valerie Hunt, to name just a few—who initially risked their reputations, have become outspoken about their holistic convictions. These people have successfully combined science and spirituality in their careers and are now widely respected and even admired for expressing such views.

There are different ways to understand the body, the human being, our existence, and our purpose here. We can look at them from a strictly physical perspective—according to Darwin's theory of evolution, we are by and large merely adaptive coincidences. But embracing a more complete and complex picture of us as spiritual beings in a physical body expands the interpretation of our purpose in a deeply satisfying and meaningful way.

Each of these perspectives offers a different definition of *health*, because each is based on a different way of understanding the body. The material view leads to a bio-physical interpretation of the body, from which arose conventional Western allopathic medicine, which treats the body essentially like a machine. According to this mechanical view, body parts can be fixed independently from one another and the rest of the human being—the cardiologist fixes your heart, the podiatrist your feet, and the internist your organs. A holistic view, on the other hand, leads to a more complete and complex spiritual or energetic interpretation of the body, from which arose Eastern and alternative medical treatment systems that regard body, mind, and spirit as an all-inclusive whole. Take stress as an example of the intricate connection between mind and body. Stress comes from excessive mental pressure we put on ourselves. Ultimately, stress boils down to fear (I read somewhere that you can reduce all emotions down to two—fear and love). If you are stressed at work, the fear might boil down to the fear of losing your job if you did what you really wanted to do, like going home on time to take care of your family or your own well-being, or telling your boss what you really think of him. Or you might be buckling under financial strain, an underlying fear of not having enough money to maintain your social standing. All fears have to do with the anxiety of potentially losing the ability to fulfill particular emotional needs, in this case the need for material safety, respect, and recognition. I will elaborate on these needs in Chapter 7, when I consider relationships and communication.

In the stress example, the connection between the spiritual and the physical is quite obvious. To relieve stress, you need to either change your beliefs and values (understanding what need your boss's irritating behavior came from, or accepting that working overtime is a fact of life in your particular job), or meeting your needs in a different way (working part-time and settling for less money, or looking for a different job). When your head tells you one thing (*I must have a "decent" job and earn so much*), and your heart tells you another (*I need more time for myself or my family*, or *I would rather work in a totally different field*), you as a person don't function in harmony because head and heart pull in different directions. Hence the stress, which vanishes once your emotional needs are met. Then body, mind, and spirit operate in unison. But when you ignore your heart's message, stress in the long run expresses itself in the physical body in the form of headaches, high blood pressure, heart problems, and can eventually even kill in form of a heart attack. The connection between mind, body, and spirit is clear here. They are inextricably linked, and we need to include this understanding in our expanded definition of health.

To summarize, two views of the human body, and of Man in general, currently co-exist in Western culture. The more prevalent, though incomplete, less complex, and outdated, one is the bio-physical interpretation of the body as a mechanism. Luckily, the more complex and complete holistic model of a body-mind-spirit organism, is on the rise. Between now and the end of Part One, I will expand the definition of what *healthy* means even further, so you will see the grander connection between health, healing, and deep living, and the gist of this book. In the meantime, here is why we currently have two models of the human being, a mechanistic and a holistic one, why this creates such stress in our culture, and why the mechanistic model is no longer adequate and satisfactory.

How Adam and Eve are related to the scientific worldview in the West

Though Isaac Newton himself, to whom we owe our scientific methods and outlook, was a deeply religious man, our culture has come to think of science and religion as incompatible. And while the Big Bang Theory may be our most recent scientific creation story, the intrinsic message of the story of Adam and Eve, our original creation story, is still deeply embedded in our cultural thinking. In a mystical and symbolic way, creation stories set root beliefs, transmit fundamental values from one generation to the next, and shape culture. The main message Western culture retains from the story of Adam and Eve's expulsion from paradise for eating from the tree of knowledge is that Heaven is good and spiritual, and Earth is not so good and not so spiritual. Bluntly put, Earth is punishment or Hell, and Heaven is paradise and a reward for good behavior. Hence our perceived disconnect from spirit, because we think of spirit as in Heaven, not on Earth. In Part Three, I will expand on another possible reason for the rift between physical and spiritual, the evolution of our consciousness. Meanwhile, let's realize that other cultures are based on other creation stories. But back to the spiritual–physical rift.

The Western creation story established the core belief that earthly life is a chore, if not worse, and that only God's grace, which cannot be counted on, only hoped for, can save us from Hell and provide us with the hope for a better predicament after death. Partly because of our particular creation story, the religions that arose from it (Judaism, Christianity, and Islam) regard Heaven and Earth, health and illness, good and bad, desirable and undesirable, spiritual and physical, male and female, and all other opposites, as contradictory and mutually exclusive and exclusionary. This has misled us to separate the material from the spiritual realm and see them as distinct. Mainstream thinking tends to see illness disconnected from wellness, as a misfortune that strikes unlucky people at random and for which they are not responsible, while the lucky ones, who have been blessed by God's grace, heal. This core belief understandably leaves us feeling helpless. Illness is not our fault, we are taught to believe. And because it puts illness outside us, we interpret it as being inflicted by an outside agent. We call this outside agent *pathology*, an external agent that we believe makes us ill. This may be a virus, bacterium, or accident-inflicted injury. Afflictions of an environmental nature, such as radiation induced sickness, or ill effects from environmental toxins, constitute a complex issue that merits a longer discussion elsewhere. But they could certainly be approached, and remediated, from an understanding of humans as part of super-organism Earth that stresses we are in it together and are all mutually responsible for the environmental damage our common cultural values have created.

The black-and-white belief system of seemingly contradictory opposites also manifests in other areas. In agriculture, for example, we eradicate pests and weeds, the supposedly undesirable outside agents, with poisons. Nutrition tries to identify *good* foods and *bad* foods, and analyzes their minute components to isolate the *good* from the *bad* nutrients. We are just awakening, for example, from the incorrect and simplistic belief that cholesterol and fats are *bad*. Many other such examples abound. Eastern philosophies, by comparison, regard opposites as belonging to the *same integrated whole*. The example of day and night is an easy one to understand. The idea of *day* only exists through its opposite, *night*. Without the concept of *night* (or darkness), there can be no such thing as *day* (or light) on Earth. As the sun comes up in the morning, night gradually gives way to day; as daylight fades, night sets in. Each is always somewhere along the way of becoming its own opposite. The familiar yin–yang symbol shows this mutually inclusive relationship by way of the white dot in the black field, and the black dot in the white field. Buddhists consider body and spirit two aspects of the same whole, leading to a different, holistic interpretation of health and illness, and of the world in general. In the West, by the way, our perception of the world used to be more holistic in earlier times, a fact I will consider further in Part Three.

Erector-set reality, or the mechanical Newtonian worldview

A first sub-belief that arose from the belief of being separated from the spiritual is the conviction that the world is strictly physical. This belief culminated during the Age of Enlightenment, in Newtonian mechanical physics and the Cartesian split of mind from matter, to establish a world picture that overrode the earlier more mystical understanding of the middle ages and led to modern science and scientific thinking, an important and essential addition to our consciousness tool box. On the other hand, science fooled us into the giddy and arrogant illusion that we could finally understand all of Nature's secrets by delving into its ever smaller parts and details. We believed that this knowledge held the key to understanding, manipulating, controlling, and transcending Nature, and to improving it to our advantage. The scientific-mechanical worldview, though, is limited, as it focuses strictly on what we can see, feel, hear, taste, and smell; all else is not considered real—*all else* being the unseen, energetic, quantum, or consciousness aspect of life.

How does this relate to health and body? From Newtonian physics emerged a mechanistic way of thinking about the world in general, and a view of the body as an Erector Set of body parts and components each of which could supposedly be repaired (aka healed) independently and out of context from the whole. Moreover, since we hoped to find the body's secrets in its ever more minute physical and biochemical details, we developed ever more specialized medical disciplines. It is understandable that such a belief system produces a different definition of health, and a different strategy for healing, than an integral body-mind-spirit belief system.

Let's improve on Nature

The second sub-belief that arose from our belief in the separatedness of the spiritual-energetic from the physical is that Nature is imperfect, and that technology lets us *improve* it. Author Charles Eisenstein dead-panned that, in an extreme case, "the ultimate victory of the Technological Program would be to triumph over death itself," which is what cryonics, for example, is hoping for.

In that context it is striking to notice the suppression of death in our culture. Since this relates directly to how we understand health and illness, let me examine it in greater detail. While many people may be religious or consider themselves spiritual, Westerners do not necessarily believe in the immortality of the soul and are thus terrorized by the supposed or potential finality of death. When death is perceived as final, illness is a reminder of death and the fragility of life. In our culture, we sweep death under the rug by avoiding confrontation with it and worshiping youth instead. Even our language reflects this ambiguous, or rather adversarial and combative, relationship with illness and death. We speak of "fighting illness and death," of "battling cancer," and "conquering a disease." We have been attempting to conquer illness with technology, and our life expectancy is proof of it. Or is it? Doctors can now prolong life by many technical means, when the body might otherwise have checked out long ago. But what if keeping a loved one in a vegetative state via a feeding tube in a hospital room was more an expression of our fear of death than a true act of compassion or technological feat to be applauded?

Trying to improve on Nature with the help of technology is

all pervasive. We have been "improving" agriculture with fertilizers, pesticides, and genetically modified organisms, with the result that birds and insects have died and biodiversity has diminished, farm workers have become ill, and our food and soil are contaminated. We have "improved" our foods with the help of chemicals in the interest of increased shelf life, marketability, and, supposedly, taste, but to the detriment of our health. We have attempted to "improve" our physical health, with the help of expensive medical technologies and drugs, to the detriment of our wallets, emotional health, and dubious successes (any eradicated diseases have been replaced by other afflictions, such as pervasive depression, stress, new afflictions like AIDS/HIV, ADD and ADHD, Lyme disease, or autism, to name just a few). Science is an essential tool when put to honorable and life-enhancing use. Modern emergency medicine is an example of this, as is the development of renewable energies, molecular cuisine, or the technology behind Pandora's internet radio. But modern combat technology, genetically modified organisms, hacking and fracking, are power- and profit-driven flip sides of the use of science and technology devoid of ethical values.

Fall from the spiritual connection and our Western pathological, reactionary, and helpless ways

The final cultural manifestation of separatedness from the spiritual is our one-sided focus on the negative, the pathological. Culturally we are simply not trained to cultivate wellness. We have lost focus of the whole and see only one side. We find it easier to define illness than health. We find it easier to say what we *don't* want than what we *do*, because we are unable to see that they are two sides of the same coin. So, in our pathology-oriented culture, we specifically hone in on illness instead of health. As such, we watch with bizarre fascination on television everything we *don't* want (all sorts of disasters, our cultural problems like drug epidemics, our politicians' embarrassments). Because of this conditioning, we have an easier time defining illness than health (i.e., "health is the absence of illness").

In addition, Western culture is reactionary instead of proactive. We have let ourselves become culturally conditioned to treating physical symptoms because we are untrained to ongoing and proactive rebalancing. Take the current child obesity epidemic in America (and elsewhere). We are now reacting to the consequences of decades of unwholesome nutrition and are wondering how we wound up here. But the writing on the wall has been in plain sight ever since the massive onslaught of fast and processed foods. Elizabeth Mackenzie of the University of Pennsylvania recently confirmed this in a policy paper: "The fundamental problem in our healthcare system. . .is the neglect of low-tech strategies to prevent disease and promote health in favor of high-tech interventions to treat disease after it has arisen." I might add that we are not only ill-trained to maintain the wellness of our bodies but also to maintain social and cultural wellness.

Most importantly, too many of us have not been encouraged to imagine what we *do* want or can have. This takes some practice and some unlearning of culturally conditioned patterns, which I hope to help you with in this book.

One last point before I turn to the question of healing and deep living. Different cultures, with other creation stories, have different worldviews. Therefore, they understand health and healing differently from us. That is why health and healing are culturally defined, a vast subject fit for a book in itself—and I will pick up on it again in Chapter 8.

Chapter 3

HOW WE HEAL,
AND WHO DOES IT

What does healing mean?

WHEN MY THEN TEN-YEAR-OLD DAUGHTER blurted out during a conversation on health, "Well, then nobody is healthy, not even a doctor," she expressed what Roger Eastman meant in *The Ways of Religion*: "Human beings are, in effect, mentally and emotionally ill." We are all somewhere on the scale between total health and total illness, somewhat healthy or somewhat ill, some of us closer to one end of the spectrum, some to the other. Other than God, or an enlightened soul, no one on Earth is totally healthy, totally blissfully balanced. *Totally* ill, on the other end of the spectrum, is actually death, or the body's inability to remain alive under adverse circumstances. In fact, I read somewhere that "every death is a suicide." This suggests the idea of checking out subconsciously when we are "done" with life, that we may choose on a spiritual level that we have had enough, or did what we needed to do, and wish to go on. Vincent Frank Bedogne, the Teilhard de Chardin scholar, expresses it this way: "Death and lifespan function. . .as a mechanism to discard life's obsolete designs." It's interesting to consider the mass extinction of the dinosaurs from this perspective, or our own death as the end of this particular body's useful physical experience.

In the previous chapter I said that health can be equated with balance, and illness with imbalance. Healing is the process of getting from illness to wellness, from imbalance to balance. Put differently, we can interpret healing as the process of stripping away that which is not you, those layers and masks and lies and ailments you have created to protect yourself from being hurt emotionally. Seen this way, healing is a cleansing process. And if healing simply means rebalancing, or is a continuous and ongoing rebalancing and growth process, then healing means much more than treating an illness. Moreover, it suggests that you read your body and then rebalance *before* a physical symptom such as a tumor, a heart attack, or a broken leg (a symptom of imbalance as well) appears. Once we tune in to our bodies in a deeper way, we will pick up much slighter imbalances than the gross physical symptoms we call an illness. Going to bed early the night after staying up past midnight to finish a Power Point presentation for the office is a simple example of such self-adjustment. Healing becomes the quest for wholeness, as author Margaret Dailey concludes, or at least to become as whole as possible in this lifetime. According to this expanded understanding, healing is simply our lifelong pursuit of perfection and harmony; it is our individual journey for self-fulfillment and has nothing to do with the *medical* establishment.

Who is the healer?

Perhaps the most important question to ask next is *who* the healer is, or *whose responsibility* the healing is. While many Western doctors now recommend lifestyle changes for their heart patients, such as more exercise and a healthier diet, which require initiative and internal adjustment, most of the time Western medicine still puts the actual act of healing-as-an-intervention outside the patient and in *the doctor, the procedure, the medication.* Yet if dis-ease or illness is an imbalance in our own system, shouldn't we personally take charge of rebalancing ourselves? If the process works one way around to become ill, why should it not work the other way around to return to health? I am not discounting the fact that we may at times need assistance in jump-starting the process, especially when faced with deeper and more serious conditions, or that we do not benefit from emotional support from people around us during the healing process.

I agree with Lewis Mehl-Madrona, a Native American physician, healer, and author, that healing is an opportunity for inner transformation or growth, and that it is most effective when we take charge of the process. My homeopathic physician, Michele Galante, says, "In reality, no doctor can heal. Only the patient can heal himself, through their own desire. The ultimate help comes from one's inner self." Doctors provide only an "illusion of help," Galante says. "They do not do the healing." So doctors are only facilitators. And Valerie Hunt writes, along those lines, that "medication, surgery, rituals, supplements, and foods only facilitate the healing process." One of my good friends, who is a nurse and healer, refers to them as "props," these aids which set into motion and support the body's own inherent healing abilities. Healing itself is an internal mental process that we can activate through our intent and will power, which then manifests in the physical body. Once you decide to see a doctor, you have already established that you need to heal or rebalance yourself. But healing also requires that inner change or transformation, because it is the consciousness aspect that informs the physical body. By shifting the consciousness aspect, such as certain ingrained beliefs, you initiate a change on the physical level in your body. Simply swallowing a pill without that inner shift may not reach deep enough for complete healing to take place. Yet it is that inner shift that is often difficult to carry out, because we naturally resist change. This can delay or stall the healing process.

A few years ago, my very creative sister was unhappy in her job as an art director for a magazine publisher but resisted leaving, fearing the possibility of not finding a new job and the financial consequences of that. She kept thinking that she needed a break. Then she broke her foot, requiring surgery, several months in a wheelchair, and physical therapy. She did get her break from work but ultimately lost the job she no longer wanted. After several years of soul- searching, dabbling in catering, creating art objects and jewelry, and beginning to teach art to young children in workshops and a private school, she is now thriving as a full-time art teacher. The shift helped to heal her on a deeper level, and she is now much happier and fulfilled with this newfound talent.

So a quick answer to the initial question of who the healer is can be that in the end we ourselves are the healer. It is a bit more complex than that, though. If you subscribe to an integral world view, then you understand that we are all connected in mutually reciprocal and intertwined ways. We are embedded in our families, our cultures and our communities, and the matrix of consciousness. Hunt refers to this embeddedness when she says that we must take responsibility for our health, because our ill health also impacts the people around us. Just think of how unnerving it is for the whole family when a spouse comes home stressed and unraveled from work—and how quickly things can clear up and turn around with a bit of humor, a kiss, or a glass of wine. In that regard Mehl-Madrona stresses the importance and positive effect of togetherness in healing, whether it's the compassion, the extra time, and the personal interest a doctor takes; the caring and participation of the entire family in the healing process of a sick family member; or the village or circle of friends in aiding the sick person to see herself well again and encourage her in the process. The healing process therefore lies as much in the quality of the supportive relationship and trust between patient and doctor, as well as the surrounding community, as it rests with you individually. It therefore helps to see healing as a joint or communal matter, since we are connected through our relationships. And when our loved ones, and our community, can see this alternate reality of you as healthy and vibrant, it can influence and motivate you to revert to your original state of harmony.

To recap, the intent or will to heal needs to come from within, making you the primary healer. The healing process is strengthened through the support and intent of an external healer or doctor, a community, or a procedure. But external healers cannot heal a patient on their own. No medication, no procedure, can be effective if the patient is unwilling.

How we heal

Previously confused in regard to several contributors to the healing process, I was puzzled about the interconnections among wholesome nutrition and health, wholesome beliefs and health, and the various healing modalities and health. Influenced by the "power of positive thinking" and the many popular books on the "biology of belief," I had been wondering whether we could simply heal by shifting our mind somehow to thinking mostly wholesome thoughts— constructive thoughts that create and heal, instead of destructive thoughts and beliefs that hurt. But this would imply that we could heal by managing to create enough positive thoughts and beliefs, all the while sitting at home all day long, eating potato chips and watching television. Then I wondered whether eating wholesome foods alone could make us healthy, and questioned whether we could attribute illness simply to the ingestion of processed and pesticide-ridden foods. Or could we become healthy by merely implementing the lifestyle changes advocated by so many cutting- edge physicians, such as eating wholesome foods and getting adequate amounts of exercise and a good night's sleep? Or would regular meditation alone heal us? I would argue that a rise in awareness with improvement in any one area, say nutrition, is likely to eventually bring with it a rise in awareness in other areas, perhaps more exercise or better sleep or mental peace, which together will have a cumulative healing effect. But that is not all either.

Building on my earlier definition of health, at least three elements need balancing: body, mind, and spirit. We need to heal on all three levels. Austrian philosopher Rudolf Steiner argued that four elements make up the human being, not only body-mind-spirit, but physical body, life-force body, emotional body, and mental body. According to his teachings, the physical body remains balanced or heals through proper nutrition; the life-force body remains balanced or heals through healing modalities and medicines and expresses itself in the effectiveness of the body's intercellular communication; the emotional body remains balanced or heals through movement and expresses itself in the quality of our relationships; and the mental body remains balanced or heals through meditative work and expresses itself in wholesome beliefs and thinking. Which healing story you ultimately adopt, and whether we are dealing with three or four aspects, healing is a multi-layered affair and encompasses all areas of your life. All aspects must operate in harmony, balance, and synchronicity if you are to become whole or healthy. With this realization I am beginning to expand the definition of healing beyond the narrow medical pathological one.

In the complexity of the healing process lies the reason for people's varied responses to treatments. Although the four different aforementioned bodies inevitably interrelate and mutually influence one another, they respond to different treatment methods, and depending on which part is out of balance, different treatments may be more or less effective. The therapy may only have addressed one of several aspects that need healing. If a patient has successfully adopted a better diet, for example, but is surrounded by friends who do not share her values; if a patient has taken medication, but his beliefs are self-sabotaging; if a patient is stressed by a profession that runs counter to his longings—then the patient's healing process will stall. All these irritants, until resolved, will keep the patient from healing on a deeper level and achieving best health.

We need a better understanding of what the healing process is. How does it happen? How do we heal? What is healing? The question on *how* to achieve a state of better or best health is as old as humanity. Judging from the overall state of health of the world population, and from the ever-increasing amounts spent on healthcare, we have not applied the available answers satisfactorily. I say this because I do believe that the question has been answered. But not everyone is spiritually inclined to search for such answers, or the answers may be hard to comprehend. The mental shift may seem difficult to undertake. Or perhaps the shift becomes easier with enough collective momentum, a possibility I will explore in Part Three. These are all matters of a spiritual philosophical nature, which shows that the question of healing is in reality much deeper than the question of how your doctor can make your symptoms go away. Healing is the path of self-realization and can be approached from all angles. It is *not a medical issue per se.* Healing with the help of any of the medical disciplines is just one of many approaches. That is why there is art therapy now, and music therapy, and hippo therapy (therapy through horseback riding), and all sorts of other therapies besides all the myriad medical disciplines, Eastern, Western, and indigenous. Whatever helps to bring you back into balance, whatever brings you closer to who you are spiritually deep within, whatever helps you to strip away all that is not you, heals you and is a healing modality. As much as Western medicine would like you to believe it, and believes it itself: *There is no universal one-size-fits-all, guaranteed, and foolproof therapy!*

Each person's circumstances and personal history are entirely unique, and because each person is embedded in her cultural and personal belief system, the healing mode ought to be entirely custom tailored. Mehl-Madrona confirms that "healing is an individual phenomenon. Everyone does it differently. Which means that we need to study how people transform, instead of seeking what cures them." We need to figure out how to mobilize each individual's inherent healing capacities.

In the West we have been looking for safety through predictability, and we believe in standard applications. But, as Mehl-Madrona argues, "Healing is difficult to understand because it lies outside the cause-and-effect paradigm of classical mechanics."

Is the answer then that there is no particular answer? The answer is that there is no one-size-fits-all treatment for any illness, dis-ease, or imbalance. Science and the current medical establishment operate from within a specific belief system in which exceptions to the norm, whether they are of the spontaneous-healing kind, or of the some-cancer-patients-respond-to-chemotherapy-and-others-die kind, are not acknowledged for what they are: an invitation to revisit our understanding of how individuals can best mobilize their innate healing powers, and the fact that our scientific parameters of applying the same treatment for a specific set of symptoms do not always yield the same predictable outcome. You are not a statistic! You are a totally unique individual.

Healing is a spiritual thing and an individual thing. As unforgiving as this may sound at first, it leaves you and me personally responsible for our imbalances, and personally responsible for figuring out how to heal. Especially in America there has been a cultural tendency for shirking responsibility and not wanting to hear the truth. Many prefer to blame others—for slipping on an icy

sidewalk (the homeowner didn't sweep and salt the sidewalk prop-
erly, forgetting your own clumsiness, or that you were on the
phone and didn't see the icy patch); for burning yourself on a hot
paper cup of coffee (McDonald's paper cups are too thin, though
you yourself let the cup slip); for becoming overweight (it's the fast
food industry's fault, disregarding the freedom to choose what you
buy and eat); for this country's indebtedness (it's the problem of
government policies, not admitting that you, too, have lived beyond your means). Yet owning this responsibility can be exciting
and empowering. Instead of this adopted helplessness, of waiting
passively for some doctor's appointment, some treatment, the
government, or winning the lottery, it feels good to pull yourself
up by your bootstraps and just do it. Take charge!

Different culture, different reality—healing is a story

What health and healing mean is a cultural story. If the story
changes, the reality changes. Authors Larry and Lauri Fahlberg
point out that Eastern cultures see health and healing differently
from us. In broad strokes, Eastern philosophies and health models
are proactive and strive to maintain health or wellness, understood
as bodily and spiritual balance, through the regular practice of such
mental and energetic techniques as meditation, qi-gong, or tai-chi,
to name just a few. These models are wellness-oriented because
they regard the human being as a body-mind-spirit continuum or
energetic organism, a view that integrates life and death, and wellness and illness, into a holistic philosophy where neither illness
nor death have to be fought, controlled, or eradicated. Instead, illness, as the flip side of wellness, is considered an opportunity for

rebalancing in order to achieve a state of wholeness again.

Dr. Mehl-Madrona, whose healing approach is cultural context oriented, argues that, if the patient is not convinced of the doctor's "healing story," she won't follow the treatment. He believes that healing does not depend on the method or technology, but instead on the correlation between the patient's and the doctor's *stories*, which means that, as long as you believe in the same healing method your doctor does, you can heal. If you and your doctor are convinced that chemotherapy is the very best and only way to heal your cancer, then there is a strong possibility you will benefit from that therapy. Personally, I believe that chemotherapy frequently poisons and weakens the body and hinders the chances of recovery, which means that chemotherapy might not be the best choice of treatment for *me*.

Healing is a complex, multi-layered, and individual process

Valerie Hunt's perspective on health and healing is holistic as well. She, too, regards the perceived opposites of health and illness as two sides of the same coin, which clarifies the connection between health, healing, and holistic living. Hunt implies, in her definition of health, the continual and automatic self-adjustments we make, the continual dynamic and integral interaction between health and illness, balance and imbalance: "Perhaps the best measure of health is an organism which is constantly self-healing. Here, healing implies an elimination of the disturbance and maintenance of the body's integrity. . . . All healing is a movement towards wholeness with cells regenerating along their original healthy plan." In that way illness can be understood as the body's own self-adjustment mechanism to recreate balance and harmony in an effort to be whole or healed. After all, a fever—as an observable physical symptom of illness—for example, is nothing more than the body's mechanism to overcome the virus behind it through elevating the body temperature beyond the virus's ability to survive. As such, illness is the body's balancing act, compensating for a temporary deficiency in an attempt to recreate harmony, where illness and health become part of the same integral model of wholeness.

In life we continually strive for harmony, though many of us don't know it. When we are not successful in pulling through with needed adjustments to reestablish complete harmony or balance, our bodies let us know. Stress, for example, is the body's attempt to initiate the reestablishment of harmony. It signals that there is an imbalance, that something is not working for you, and that you need to change that disturbance in your life in order to reestablish harmony and rid yourself of the stress.

Over the years I have learned to listen to my body's signals and to reestablish balance right away. As I am writing this, I am on a juice fast. A few days ago, my body signaled me that an overindulgence in too much meat and fat over the summer, and a lack of greenies, are not beneficial for my digestive system. I have gained a few pounds, some of my pants are too tight, and I simply feel stuffed. I know what kind of diet is beneficial to my own digestive system but have ignored it over the past few weeks. After all, I love food, and much of my eating is for pleasure and entertainment. But enough is enough; back to a better diet, back to more exercise, back to balance.

A holistic life is a healing life, a life on the way to wholesome-ness, a life that is in harmony with who you are. The few basic universal spiritual needs we all have in common are love, respect, compassion, and trust (the physical ones are food, shelter, rest, and sex). I believe that if each of us, not only lived our personal lives in an effort to fulfill those needs wholeheartedly from a place of love, but also respected everyone else's right to do the same, the world would be a fairer, safer, and socially more just place.

Power of the mind

"It is clear that patterns of thought and emotions trigger specific illness," Valerie Hunt writes. When no one believed that AIDS could be healed as the crisis arose in the 1980s, the effect was the same as the voodoo condemnation to death in which a condemned person literally dies from a combination of the community's mental conditioning and her own fear. A recent scientific study has documented how several patients with arthritic knees healed successfully after undergoing placebo surgery, surgery they thought had happened when in fact it had not. And a study on people with multiple personality disorder revealed diabetic symptoms in one study subject while inhabiting one of her personalities, but not when she switched to a different personality, which illustrates the incredible influence our mind and beliefs have on our physical condition.

A quarter-century after the AIDS crisis began, things have changed dramatically, and AIDS has shifted from a death sentence to a manageable chronic illness, because the underlying belief system has shifted and no longer discounts the possibility of survival. As soon as one person lives longer than expected, the possibility of survival begins to exist for all of us, and others follow suit. When you break a leg or get a sore throat, you take it for granted that you will heal, and you recognize the cast or the cup of hot tea as props that support the body in its healing process. You would never attribute the cast or the hot tea to the healing itself. However, when it comes to what we consider *serious* or *incurable* diseases, we tend to change the rules and let beliefs get in the way. All of a sudden, we believe otherwise, that it is the *medication* that causes the healing. And that makes all the difference. This collective- belief phenomenon has also been observed in regard to world records in sports. Sometimes a world record remains unbroken for years. Yet as soon as that record is broken, several people are able to meet or exceed it shortly thereafter.

As Bruce Lipton puts it in *The Biology of Belief*, "The brain *controls* the behavior of the body's cells." He means that our own minds are responsible for a large part of our mental balance or imbalance, which in turn creates the biology of the cells, or their pathology. While mind power is thus responsible for much of our well-being or our dis-ease, health is a complex matter, and mind power alone is unlikely to heal us by itself if we don't provide the body with favorable conditions.

Why so many different ways to heal?

There are as many different ways to heal as there are people. The many different modalities initially arose from different cultural perspectives. We all heal in our own ways.

These approaches don't, by any means, have necessarily to be *medical*, as I showed earlier. In addition, as long as we look to the

outside for solutions to the lessening of our suffering or to fulfillment—to doctors, to medical procedures and medications, to miracle diets, to winning the lottery, and so on—we may only have
limited success. The more we look for solutions inside ourselves,
and the more we shed everything that is "not us," as Dr. Galante
puts it, the better we heal.

Broadening the concept of healing to understand it as the
search for who we are is a leap I made when I searched for definitions of health and healing during one of my graduate courses. I
have attempted to show that healing is so much more than getting
rid of symptoms, and that the bio-medical definition of healing is
too narrow. Life is self-realization through interaction with people
and our environment. Thus, healing is the realization of our
human potential, of finding fulfillment and oneness with the spiritual from within. I understand healing as the journey of finding
myself, my innermost who-I-really-am. It involves gradually shedding everything I am not, and moving further and further away
on the wellness spectrum from illness and imbalance, and closer
and closer to well-being and self-realization.

One last thought: Although there are medical cases of spontaneous remission or spontaneous healing, and cases of sudden
enlightenment, healing in most cases is a gradual process. We do
so in stages, climbing up a ladder so to speak. And because everything on the spiritual level is interconnected within us and around
us, any healing or rebalancing in one area of ourselves has an effect
on all other areas. If you heal your relationship with food, how
you eat and what you eat, as we will explore in Chapter 6, your relationships with the soil, the Earth, and your body are likely to
change, and vice versa—by tending to a vegetable garden, you are

likely to reevaluate your relationships with food, your body, and
Nature. If you heal the way you communicate with people, as we
will investigate in Chapter 7, your relationships will inevitably shift
and heal.

Many times a trigger experience or event initiates such a shift.
My relationship with food gradually changed after my children
were born. Wanting to feed my babies only the very best out of
deep love and the need to protect them, I began to become aware
of, and started to research, the food realities of our times. Gradually I converted to organics, beginning with dairy, then expanding
to fruits, vegetables, and grains, and finally to meats and fish. My
awakening is ongoing, and my food awareness went through a further shift after my daughter was diagnosed with Type 1 Diabetes
last year.

Taking charge, and how healing and holistic living relate

When I am not well, which happens quite rarely, my husband
gets all flustered, because it affects the family balance so much.
All of a sudden, so many things that are taken for granted don't
get taken care of. Therefore, if *I* heal, everyone and everything
around me heals with me. Think of a drop of water falling into a
puddle. It forms concentric circles that reverberate out and out
and out, far beyond the original size and energy of the droplet.
When you bloom, everyone around you blooms with you.

I have defined healing as a rebalancing of imbalances, or as living true to your heart. I have also said that the healer is ultimately
no one but yourself. You and I are in charge! And that is actually
a good thing, because why would I want someone else to decide

what is good for me? I am the creator of my life. I am the healer of my life. What is *your* storyboard?

A holistic life is an awakened life

A holistic life incorporates both the material and spiritual aspects of your existence. While we perceive the physical aspect with our five senses, we delve into the spiritual part with our consciousness and heart. Our emotions and feelings are a barometer of this aspect. By embracing that *other* part, life becomes balanced. We no longer simply ask *how much* and *how fast*, we also ask *how well*. This aspect adds significance and meaning to life; it adds layer, depth, and quality. A life without it is dead. Balancing heals you both mentally and physically. A holistic life is a sustainable life that works in harmony with Nature, our fellow beings, and the highest good for all. Moreover, because a holistic life is non-competitive, it is a win-win for all. It is a participatory life lived in awareness. It is a creative life, and it is beneficial for all, not just for some. Therefore, it becomes a sustainable and socially just way of life. Social change and justice, a greener planet, a sustainable life, and self-fulfillment all begin with you and me. Holistic living is a wake-up call.

Perhaps now you are ready to heal specific areas of life, your relationships with Nature, agriculture, food, your body, and others. This is what we'll explore in Part Two.

PART TWO

Reinventing Our Connections

Chapter 4

MAN AS PART OF NATURE, NOT APART FROM NATURE

"You did not weave the web of life, you are a mere strand in it. Whatever you do the web, you do to yourself."

—*Chief Seattle (c. 1780–1866)*

Introduction

DEEP LIVING ENTAILS A DEEPER AWARENESS OF, and involvement with, everything that pertains to our everyday life, and so it does with our relationship to Nature. "The Great Indoors" is how author Charles Eisenstein refers to our era, and I can relate to that, because I mainly grew up indoors in big cities. Though we now live in the country, my daughter's school has indoor recess when it rains, and when the temperature rises above 85°F many of us switch our air-conditioners on and stay indoors. Many suburbanites want their lawns weed-free or panic when little slugs munch on the lettuce in their vegetable patch, to which they generally prefer quick solutions in a spray can.

What does all of this say about our relationship with Nature?

Many of the Western cultural beliefs we visited in Part One influence how we generally think about Nature and how people interact with it (or not). I showed in Part One that those predominant beliefs are just that, not facts, and that they can and will change with the ongoing evolution of our consciousness, the way beliefs have always historically evolved (after all, people did at one point firmly believe the Earth was flat). In the case of our relationship with Nature, these beliefs are the cause of our present environmental nightmare.

In this chapter I will introduce some thoughts and consciousness trends as inspiration for a new and improved relationship with Nature to help us heal the Earth. Before that, though, let's take a quick excursion into our present relationship with our surroundings in order to place the alternative beliefs and thought movements into perspective.

Our love-hate relationship with Nature, and why we think Nature is so scary

Generally speaking people want a happy life in a beautiful world. Nonetheless, it is striking that much of Nature no longer looks so beautiful, whether we are thinking about Beijing's air pollution, the logged Amazonian rain forest, the nightmarishly large plastic swirls in the Pacific Ocean, or the fast food plastic cup someone thoughtlessly threw out their car window onto the roadside. It is slowly dawning on some of us that *we* did the damage, collectively.

Although there are other, more eco-centric, traditions, many of them indigenous, the world's three main religions, which have shaped our Western thinking, have all spawned anthropocentric cultures. These regard us humans as the central purpose of earthly existence and place us apart from, and in a superior position to, other natural elements and beings. Many indigenous people, on the other hand, still, literally, live close to Nature (nearer the ground than we in our skyscrapers) and gather or grow some or all of their food themselves, which creates a more symbiotic, aware relationship with Nature. But to most of us city dwellers in industrialized countries, Nature has become a somewhat abstract concept. While things are also changing for indigenous people, they have traditionally believed in the sacredness of their surroundings, that Nature is somehow alive, and that it nurtures them. Therefore they have lived in a cooperative and respectful relationship with Nature, adopted what we might call a *stewardship* of the environment. Don't misunderstand me here. This is not about idolizing indigenous people and calling for our return to the woods; it's about maturing beyond our present stage. In Part Three, I will address evolutionary consciousness stages, which may help to approach the indigenous mind from a more differentiated perspective.

For the rest of us, that sacred relationship with Nature started to crumble after the middle ages and disappeared with industrialization, when the belief emerged that Earth is a storehouse of gold, oil, gas, and minerals we can loot. With increasing urbanization, most of us lost the realization of the intricate web-like relationship and interdependence between Man and the world he inhabits. Eventually, this loss led us to reclassify some elements of Nature, such as certain insects (which we now call pests), plants (which we now call weeds), floods, forest fires, and droughts as flaws or nuisances that we can improve or fix with technologies like pesticides, herbicides, and damming. Nature has become an abstract *out there* for our garbage, too. It is only very slowly dawning on us that our surroundings are like a house of cards, and that we are sitting inside it. Removing just one card from somewhere in the middle of the house causes it to collapse. When we spray crops against just one particular insect, for example, the whole food chain becomes imbalanced, and the consequences reverberate out and out. *Though not all of us see the Spirit in Nature, that doesn't mean it's not there.*

Growing up in big cities, I had no connection to the outdoors besides some Sunday walks in the park. Nor did I have a connection to the hamsters, guinea pigs, and fish of my childhood apartment existence. Friends' sniffing and licking dogs were an annoyance I bore stoically. How things have changed. I love our adorable cats unconditionally. I just cannot be upset with them, even when they scratch up the leather dining room chairs. And I enjoy the loving cat kisses from their sweet little rough and pink tongues. Our cats have taught me to see the inner beauty and perfection in any animal. I am sad when I see a deer on the side of the road that has been run over, and I cringe when a squirrel runs out in front of my car and scream for it to get out of the way. Physicist and Sufi initiate Thomas Maxwell has said, "True compassion is born when we realize that the same divine light that shines through our own being also shines through all other sentient beings." Such a change in belief and behavior is no longer driven by moralistic coercion but comes from within. The same goes for our relationship with the rest of Nature. When the heart opens up to our complete dependence on it, Nature's beauty shines through in gratefulness, and we become incapable of mindlessly throwing a candy wrapper away on a hike in the woods. For fear of getting stung, I used to wave my arms around as soon as I saw a bee in the far distance—which is actually more likely to incite a bee to sting you. Since we have kept bees, I have learned that bees are really docile, that they get to know those who care for them, and that they only sting when they feel threatened, not least because they actually lose their life after that one sting, unlike wasps that can sting multiple times.

We fear the unknown, and Nature has become unknown to many of us. Because we live apart from it, we can find it unsettling or downright dangerous. To compensate, we want to control it, dominate it, and make it predictable, which we attempt to do with the help of technology. In ignorance of other methods, or impatience with methods that may take longer, we spray herbicides to control the weeds on the lawn, pesticides to kill the little critters on the lettuce, or dam rivers to control flooding. Nature is forgiving and constantly adjusts and rebalances. That's why it usually takes a few decades to really encounter the consequences of our interference, whether they are dying bats and bees (likely due to immune-weakening pesticides and the industrial handling of bee colonies for the pollination of large orchards), human-induced climate change and more extreme weather patterns (as a consequence of fossil fuel and methane emissions, and the disappearance of large swaths of rain forest due to logging), or mutated salmon (due to genetic modification), to name just a few.

The connection between The Economy and Nature

Buying your eggs from your local sustainable farmer instead of supermarket eggs from battery-cage chickens for less than half

the price makes all the difference, because Nature and the economy are so closely related. But the relationship has grown so abstract nowadays that it is difficult to see. We may have forgotten
that everything we need to live comes from Nature, instead believing it comes from *The Economy*, as environmentalist, geneticist,
and author David Suzuki points out. Yet whether it is our food (although I have heard that some city children believe that food
comes from the supermarket, and big food would have us believe
that it comes from factories), gold, coal, minerals, fiber for making
clothes, or timber for building homes, everything we need to make
something comes from the Earth. If it weren't for Nature, we'd
have no economy; heck, we wouldn't exist. Once we come to that
realization, we'll treat Nature again with reverential gratitude and
respect. *Without Nature we would not exist.*

Suzuki remarks that we have made ourselves the slaves of *The
Economy*, in whose name we are "monoculturing the planet with a
single notion of progress and development that is embodied in the
globalized economy." Ever since colonialism, we have felt superior
in the Great Western Way of thinking and have erroneously believed that environmental concern is linked to development and
affluence. We project our economic-materialist worldview onto
Third World and *developing* countries (both heavily loaded terms)
in the misconstrued conviction that they won't be able to cultivate
environmental concerns until their yearning for the trappings of
our material culture have been satisfied. But that belief may be
based simply on our lack of an alternative vision. Examination of
indigenous cultural values and the present state of affairs in the
Western world has shown that self-realization is what makes us
happy, and that happens through relationships and doing the

things we like to do. As *New York Times* reporter Stephanie Rosenbloom has written, "Academics are already in broad agreement that there is a strong correlation between the quality of people's relationships and their happiness." So it is not the chase for wealth and material accumulations that makes us happy and fulfilled. *Happiness is unrelated to material wealth.*

The ultimate problem with our material-capitalistic system, however, is that it is based on continuous growth and the perceived need to make more tomorrow than today because—well, you never know. Continuous growth borrows from the future; it is based on credit (buy now, pay later) and on an economics of scarcity. We switched to this type of thinking as a consequence of evolving from a nomadic to a settled lifestyle (which was a result of our evolving consciousness—more on this in Part Three). A nomadic lifestyle permits Nature to renew itself after a group of people has passed through an area and harvested its food. In a settled or urban lifestyle, people live in the same area year-in and year-out, so we invented agriculture to feed ourselves. With agriculture came two challenges. One is that the environment immediately surrounding the settlement does not renew itself on its own. The other is that the area surrounding a settlement is limited, and becomes more limited if the population grows and requires more food. From this situation arose the belief that there is never enough. This illusion of scarcity encouraged a tendency to accumulate more than we require for our immediate future.

The solution to overcoming our present economic model is not, however, to paddle backwards and return to a nomadic lifestyle. Evolution is always about moving forward and maturing creatively, enhancing life along the way, and furthering ourselves.

We take the essence of the past with us and build on it, rendering life more complex, more diverse, more creative, and perhaps more spiritual. Ideas for the renewal of our economic system go beyond the scope of this book, but two of its most eloquent visionaries are Jeremy Rifkin and Charles Eisenstein.

What Darwin did to our relationship with Nature

Social Darwinism, an extension of Darwin's theory of natural selection of stronger organisms through gradual functional adaptation, emerged in conjunction with capitalism and evolved into the theory of survival through competition, conflict, and winning of the fittest. This thinking is deeply ingrained in us culturally. Linking this to thoughts about economic scarcity results in the message that there is not enough, so we have to fight for the little there is, and that the fitter survive and the weaker perish. Moreover, if only the tough, quick, and ruthless survive, sharing is not an option, although David Sloan Wilson has argued altruism from a Darwinian perspective. In that regard, philanthropy in this country is not necessarily a sign of generosity and compassion but, first and foremost, driven by tax incentives. The philosophy of scarcity perpetuates the belief that we need to produce more today in order to have enough for tomorrow (squirrel it away, and don't share it), and to buy today (and pay later) because tomorrow there may not be anything left (the Black Friday phenomenon). Save for college, save for retirement, save for a rainy day, buy insurance for everything—life, disability, house, calamities that are likely never to manifest, credit monitoring, what have you. We spend so much money on insurance, whether in the form of various types of savings or insurance policies, that we live a little less for it. We simply cannot fathom that the universe will always provide for us.

In our present cultural universe of unrelated opposites (darkness as the opposite of light instead of the other *aspect* of light, without which light is not possible, and as a fluid spectrum that goes to and fro between both aspects), we exist in parallel realities from Nature's elements, as *other* than Nature, as separate from it and superior. This belief is behind our acts of poisoning and sullying our planet, because the planet, Nature, the surrounding environment, *seem* other. Yet a different underlying belief system, a holistic one, would allow for a more reverential and co-operative relationship with Nature, because we would see ourselves as an integral part of it.

A beautiful example of such a holistic relationship that has successfully operated for hundreds of years is that of the Balinese rice growers David Suzuki cites. These people live in a profoundly symbiotic relationship with Nature, religion, agriculture, and neighboring people that is based on a deep awareness and appreciation of the web-like interrelationships among the various elements of their existence. As in my earlier house-of-cards analogy, the alteration of any one component in this fine balance affects the entire system, a complex system that can only be maintained by insiders who are aware of all the conditions and factors. Suzuki reports that the system actually *did* collapse for a period of time when arrogant Western scientists imposed genetically modified rice and Western agricultural practices on those indigenous rice growers in an ill-guided attempt to "improve" conditions. The balance was subsequently reestablished, and the scientists learned their lesson, albeit at the expense of a painful decade or two for the rice growers.

I am now ready to move beyond framing our present relationship with Nature. The environmental movement of the 1970s, with its awakening to the damage we have inflicted on Nature, also opened our awareness to the question of how to live with it for our mutual benefit. A variety of inspirational movements and concepts now promote a harmonious, co-creative, non-adversarial, and non-competitive relationship with our surroundings. It is no coincidence that many of their premises overlap, and that all point in the same general direction.

Deep Ecology and self-realization

Deep Ecology stands for a deeper-than-common interpretation of ecology. Norwegian philosopher Arne Naess's Deep Ecology movement was born in the 1970s out of a rising environmental awareness. Its central idea is self-realization or self-fulfillment for all and everything. This means giving humans, animals, plants, rocks, insects, the cosmos, everyone and everything, the opportunity to be the best they can be, or the "opportunity for perfection," as Teilhard de Chardin scholar Frank Bedogne puts it. For one, this idea promotes a non-anthropocentric, co-operative, deeply respectful, and compassionate relationship with Nature, which regards all entities of the Earth as equally important, as mutually beneficial and reciprocally interrelated, and which interact by way of continuous adjustment and rebalancing. This latter idea is very similar to the way Valerie Hunt described the human healing process, as I explained in Chapter 3.

Like Thomas Maxwell, Naess noticed that a progression in self-realization, what I call self-fulfillment, deepening spirituality, or consciousness awakening, automatically brings with it a deepening connection to all living beings and the environment. Over the years, my relationship with plants, for example, has changed. When I walk through my vegetable garden, I get a real thrill out of watching sprouts emerging from seeds in the soil and their gradual growth into mature vegetable plants. Although it happens the same way every year, each year I take pictures anew of the rows of lush vegetables, because I am in awe of the beauty and abundance and magic of how this happens so naturally (pun intended) yet seems to be such a complex and amazing process. Watching this emergence of life unfold is enormously meaningful and, I dare say, spiritual. In that regard Naess has observed that many followers of Deep Ecology are vegetarians, a development others also see in conjunction with deepening spirituality. But Naess's philosophy goes further yet and overlaps with many spiritual paths. He maintains that ever-increasing self-realization for all of Nature's entities (us included) entails ever-increasing diversity (it's not interesting to have a Starbucks on every corner), ever-increasing complexity (in opposition to simplification; nervous systems, for example, are more complex the more developed and complicated an organism is), ever-increasing co-operation and symbiosis (interdependencies, in which all partners are enriched, a "no man-is-an-island" mentality), increasing local autonomy and decentralization (local stewardship and empowerment), and increasing equal rights and social justice. The implications of these premises are not only a movement towards radical social change, which is how Naess put it, but an evo-

lution towards higher consciousness and greater spiritual awareness.

TEK and native wisdom

We have come a long way from the condescending colonial attitude towards native societies and are beginning to recognize that
indigenous people have a lot to teach us. Native cultures' holistic
relationship with Nature is a true source of inspiration. I became
interested in this other cultural reality when I read with fascination anthropologist Carlos Castaneda's famous books about the
teachings of the Mexican shaman Don Juan. While we have gained
a lot from the Age of Enlightenment, namely science and scientific
thinking, we have (temporarily, I believe) lost our sense of the sacred and the spiritual, believing that the two are incompatible,
and that one is superior to the other. To indigenous people, Nature is alive, since something dead, something devoid of consciousness, cannot be sacred. Sacredness means capable of being
worshiped because inhabited by spirit. Native cultures, writes
David Barnhill, a professor of environmental studies, derive their
"sacred truth from Nature not scripture," in contrast to us. That
is an important observation suggestive of the differences between
cosmologies. Indigenous people live an integral holistic reality—
Barnhill calls theirs the "undivided Native mind"—although contact with Western culture compromises that.

Four native concepts, all mentioned by David Suzuki, help inspire us towards a better relationship with Nature—cooperation,
localism or decentralization, circularity, and patience. These ideas
are worthwhile examining in detail.

A. Co-operation:

Indigenous cultures center around community and are co-operative. Within their belief system, Man is not superior to any other part of Nature but an equal and integral part of it. We are not islands, but exist through a web of relationships with family, friends, and community on the one hand, and our environment, or Nature, on the other. Dependence has been portrayed sometimes as a sign of weakness, and at least in the U.S. we have come to regard independence as in living off the grid or, e.g., *The Lone Ranger*, as a sign of strength. In reality that is a misinterpretation. In fact, it has been shown that a *good social network is good for your health.*

And we might deduce the same about an interdependent relationship with Nature. Rituals and festivals revolve around native peoples' appreciation for Nature as a provider and sacred entity. Natives live in synchronicity with their environment and, because of their deep knowledge of the surrounding ecosystem, continuously adjust their interaction with it. This fluidity of ongoing adjustment, as opposed to resistance, is also behind Taoism's first principles and was equally well expressed by the Greek philosopher Heraclitus: "The only thing constant is change."

We will find this principle again in the next chapter when I talk about Permaculture.

The management and upkeep of the Appalachian Trail models such a respectful relationship between Man and Nature. Human impact is kept to a minimum, everyone must take their trash out with them, and the trail is rerouted whenever human impact becomes too apparent, permitting Nature to renew itself. This type of relationship is sustainable because it is based on mutual respect and appreciation.

By shifting the way we see our relationships, with Nature and with people, to co-operative and non-adversarial, we are creating win-win situations for both sides, an unusual concept in our present cultural paradigm, in which we tend to believe that one party must lose for the other to win.

B. Decentralization or localism:

There has been a lot of criticism in recent years that government is out of touch with the people it governs. Indeed, the further geographically away a government operates from its constituency, the more its decisions will tend to be abstract, self-serving, or bottom-line oriented instead of executed in the best interest of local circumstances, simply because it cannot deeply know these local circumstances, conditions, and histories. Far-away governance is carried out by people without a vested interest in local matters, one of the downsides of globalization, which Suzuki defines as "perceiving the entire planet as the source of resources while all people in the world form a potential market." In fact, I recently read that the optimal nation has a population of between three and nine million people. Governments of countries with larger populations are thus out of touch with their constituents. The same principle often applies to very large corporations.

In contrast, indigenous people, those who have lived in smaller communities for generations, as well as traditional farmers, are one with their land because they have inhabited it for as long as they can remember. They identify with it and know and revere it deeply. Native cultures' local knowledge is now recognized under the acronym TEK, for traditional ecological knowledge. These people have a profound realization that their land provides them with all they need to live a good life. In this age of moving around and away from home, theirs is a symbiotic relationship with the land that is difficult for many of us to imagine. I, for one, moved away from where I was born at the age of two, and lived in many different places and countries before settling where I have been for the past twenty or so years.

From an intimate relationship with one's land naturally arises a reverential stewardship of it and a vested interest in local politics and community affairs. In addition to the awareness of total interdependence, it includes knowledge of local history and of local conditions and circumstances. Michael Northcott, Professor of Ethics at the University of Edinburgh, calls "community-based ecological politics. . .a key strategy for the renewal of democracy against those anti-democratic forces of monopoly capitalism and global bureaucracies which constantly threaten to remove control of natural resources from local people." Shifting from an attitude that declares, "It doesn't matter whether I vote or not," to becoming involved in the local community makes a big difference. The needed shift is about more than just buying American; it is about creating truly local economies in order to control the quality of life directly.

C. Circularity:

Industrial processes are in general linear. An exception is the recycling industry, which strives to bring materials back into the production process, and whose motto is "reduce, reuse, recycle." As a result, a number of products are now made from partially or totally recycled materials. Linear processes are finite in comparison to cyclical ones. We extract resources from the earth, manufacture something from them, and eventually this something becomes waste. Think of a plastic toy your toddler has outgrown and that ends up in the garbage because it is not worthy of being saved for the next generation. If the process ends there, it becomes a one-way street with a big consequence: trash and pollution. Things that can be used over and over, on the other hand, such as a glass jar or a wooden toy train, or that can be recycled, such as paper or organic waste, live a cyclical life. Aluminum, for example, can be recycled and reused indefinitely, and composted organic waste becomes fertilizer for the next round of crops. Those items do not end up in the waste stream but begin their life anew.

All natural cycles are cyclical and indefinitely repeatable without depletion of the principal or creation of waste. That is the definition of *sustainable*. The seasons are such a natural cycle, as are the planetary revolutions, or birth, life, and death (not everyone will agree here). Another example is the water cycle. The quantity of water on Earth is finite, and it changes continuously from one form into another in an eternal cycle. Suzuki points to the importance of "transforming our thinking from the linearity of extracting, processing, manufacturing, selling, using and discarding" into the circularity of natural cycles. Hence the attractiveness of renewable energy sources like solar, wind, and water power, because sun, wind, and water will always be available—the principal does not get depleted through use; whereas coal, gas, and oil are gone forever once extracted and burnt, in addition to which their combustion generates waste. Planting perennial food crops in favor of annual plants applies this circularity principle to agriculture. I will discuss its deeper benefits in more detail in the next chapter. It is a matter of awareness and priorities to develop circular processes to fulfill our needs. *A sustainable process is a cyclical process that can be repeated indefinitely without depletion of the principal or creation of waste.*

D. Patience:

Because indigenous people traditionally have trusted Nature and its abundance, as our nomadic ancestors did, they live for today, not for tomorrow. Thus there is no need to produce surplus beyond what is needed for the immediate future—no need for credit, insurance, or much storage. But we have become used to instant gratification. Information is now available at the touch of a finger. We no longer write letters but send e-mails, texts, and tweets. We can order almost anything over the internet and have it delivered within a day or two. Our attention spans have become shorter, as teachers have noticed in schoolchildren, and the movie and TV industries exploit and promote that fact, and scenes and frames become shorter and shorter to suit. On the material side, the credit system has enabled us to acquire a house or a car without paying for it up front. The principle of living on credit, banking on a better future to fulfill our needs and wants *now* and pay for it later, is also coloring our relationship with Nature. Coupled with a fear of change, many don't want to believe—yet, anyhow—that oil and natural gas reserves are finite. Many don't want to believe—yet—that we have a garbage problem. Many don't want to believe—yet—that climate change is man-made, real, here, and calamitous if not addressed immediately. Many don't want to believe that we have any number of other grave environmental problems. Technology will fix them in the future, we seem to hope on the ostrich principle (if I hide my head in the sand, I won't see the problem and can ignore it for a while longer).

Environmentally speaking, we live on credit and shirk the responsibility for cleaning up our environmental act *now*. We still look for quick solutions in a spray can. But most quick solutions have detrimental side effects in the long run. Instead of patiently deferring some of our material wants and paying for environmental clean-ups now, we pass on the dirty work and the hidden cost to our children. This is immature and plain unfair. The required shift in attitude needs to come from within each of us, *not* from The Government. The government has no choice but to follow suit when pressure from the bottom is significant enough. From indigenous cultures we need to relearn patience and a long-term approach. Ian Prattis, a professor emeritus at Ottawa's Carleton University, reminds us that Native Americans used to live by the principle of "looking ahead seven generations into the future." Being patient is about deferring the yearning for instant gratification (such as "buying now and paying later") for the greater common good, out of a mature sense of responsibility and awareness.

The Transition Movement

The Transition Movement is the last inspirational movement I am presenting as an alternative way to interact with Nature. Its

British founder, Rob Hopkins, maintains that sustainability does not go far enough, since sustainability, according to his definition, is merely about "reducing the impact" of our lifestyle and perpetuating it with the help of improved technology, as opposed to drawing the more far-reaching conclusion that we lead an untenable lifestyle based on untenable beliefs. The Transition Movement, which was founded in 2005, foresees the collapse of our unsustainable industrial economic culture due to depletion of the fossil fuels it is built upon. The movement is about proactive change from within to a new socio-economic model. It is based on the principles of permaculture—Bill Mollison and David Holmgren's principles for creating a *permanent culture*—which I will explain in more detail in the next chapter on agriculture. *New York Times* writer Jon Mooallem summarizes the Transition Movement as being about "walkable villages, local food and artisans, [and a] greater intimacy with the natural world." While it is only indirectly about a better relationship with Nature, enacting the movement's principles will naturally lead us to interact with the environment in a more vested way.

Our present global economy is based on continuous growth, which has been made possible through the enormous input of the fossil fuel energies coal, gas, and oil, energies we use to run factories, to fuel machines for businesses, agriculture, and industry, and for long-distance transportation of goods and people. But continuous growth is physically impossible because of the finite size of our planet. Due to the looming depletion of fossil fuels, the Transition Movement foresees a natural contraction after centuries of globalization and growth. While renewable energy sources may be part of the picture of our future, continuous growth, as in ever more people, ever more stuff, ever bigger homes for everyone, ever more animal protein for everyone, ever more garbage, is physically limited by the size of our planet and thus impossible.

The Transition Movement embraces the ideas of TEK and many of Naess's Deep Ecology tenets. It advocates ideas of local empowerment and self-governance, a cooperative community approach, local economies, and local land use decisions based on intimate knowledge of local conditions. In tune with Nature's inherent drive towards greater diversity and creativity, the movement does not promote a one-size-fits-all how-to prescription. Instead, it seeks to empower local entities to envision and create each community's individualized solution based on local circumstances, history, and the community's vision. There are currently 160 initiatives in North America, and 1,196 worldwide.

Is Nature intelligent?

It is easy to make fun of rain dancing or of people who say they can communicate with animals. I've already discussed the idea of spirit or consciousness bringing forth matter through a creative impulse, and that indigenous cultures worship Nature for its sacredness. Physicist F. David Peat reports that the Blackfoot Indians used to caution to "tread lightly upon Earth, for it is a living thing rather than dead matter." The question of whether Nature is intelligent is quite valid. It is a question that cautiously arose in the 1970s with James Lovelock's famous Gaia principle, the idea of Earth as a living organism.

For me this idea is neither kooky nor far-out and merits consideration. A number of scientists like Fritjof Capra, Humberto Maturana, and Francisco Varela, to name but a few, have recently explored this possibility. And an amalgam of such scientific thinking (perhaps still revolutionary to some), indigenous beliefs, and elements of the new New Physics reads something like this: Nature *is* consciousness, it doesn't *have* a consciousness. Nature is intelligent, an intelligence that is all-permeating and which we are an integral part of. We, and all of Nature and the cosmos, bring forth this reality we call Earth and our environment. Accordingly, every thing is mutually interdependent with the entire web of things. Intelligence exists in every bodily cell; it permeates everything. Peat calls this a "participatory cosmos." If we are indeed connected with all of Nature on a consciousness level, then rain dancing or communicating with animals seem less outlandish, because they are interactions on a quantum or energetic level. Part Three of this book picks up the question of intelligent life from the perspective of an evolving consciousness.

So what is Nature? And who are we in relationship to it?

From the perspective of a "participatory cosmos," or Nature as consciousness, or intelligent Nature, which we are all a part of, which we are one with, which we are interdependent with in a mutual and reciprocal relationship, Chief Seattle's alleged remark, "Whatever you do the web, you do to yourself" makes sense. The realization that we wouldn't and couldn't exist without Nature, independently from it, is powerful and causes a shift in our relationship with it. If you are still unconvinced, read Dr. Seuss's *The*

Lorax. Once we recognize this on a deeper level, we no longer have to be coerced into refraining from throwing a paper cup out of the car window (because we know we'd pollute our environment, desecrate Nature, and make someone else eventually pick up our garbage), spraying pesticides on the apple trees in the orchard (because we'd know we'd poison the bees, birds, and other plants, the groundwater, the adjacent neighbors' air, and our own bodies once we eat the apples), or throwing the batteries out with the regular garbage (because we'd know that lead in the batteries would eventually leak into the soil and groundwater, the same soil we grow our food in and the same groundwater that serves as our drinking water). We know that this would bite us in the tail, because the environment is part of us, and we couldn't possibly sully that which we depend upon for our livelihood. *Nature is life. You are it. You are Nature.*

How to connect more deeply with Nature

There are many areas where you can begin experiencing a deeper awareness of your embeddedness in Nature, and you will find the way that comes naturally to you. A psychic said to me years ago, "You need to connect more deeply with trees and plants." I bought a tree identification guide that has been sitting on my bookshelf ever since and has done nothing to help me connect more deeply with plants. The process actually worked the other way round. Once my awareness had opened up years later, vegetable gardening brought me closer to plants, and owning cats brought me closer to animals, just like that.

If you live in a big city it is more difficult to connect with

Nature, as it was for me when I grew up. But even there, you can begin your deeper relationship with pets, houseplants, or planter gardening, windowsill herbs, or the trees and the sky in the park.

Since so many people have pets, this is a good place to start. My cats taught me to see the inner beauty in any animal, where earlier I had just seen *animal* as something abstract I felt no connection to. The deep relationship with my cats opened up my awareness to the spirit in any animal. Think about what you feed your pets, how you treat them, and whether that relates to how much you appreciate them. When you look into your dog's or cat's eyes, it is not difficult to see the spirit in them and become filled with love and appreciation, which may be a bit more difficult with a turtle or guppies.

Plants are another easy way to connect with Nature, whether through flower or vegetable gardening or houseplants, windowsill herbs, or tree hugging, which is supposed to give you good energy. Watching vegetables growing from tiny dried seeds out of a packet to strong plants has been a deeply meaningful and empowering experience for me. Or nurturing an orchid through the dormant months and finally seeing a new shoot emerging from underneath the leaves, which eventually unfolds into a new flower stem beautifying my home for months, is truly special.

Hiking and wilderness experiences get you *into* Nature in a more direct way, as does farming. Several summers ago, I went camping for the first time in my adult life. The first few nights, I had trouble sleeping because I was not used to the vulnerability of sleeping outside and hearing the wind whistling in the trees or the rain drumming on the tent. It soon became a beautiful experience, though.

We did it again the next summer, and the next, and I love it.

Get your children off their screens and outside. My daughter used to say, "But what do I *do* out there? There's nothing to *do*." Then she found a friend who shared her love for the outdoors, and now they always find things to make and do. My husband built our daughter a lean-to where she used to sit with her friend, chatting and watching the stream flow by.

If you're interested in politics, consider getting involved in local land use or environmental matters in your community.

You might consider installing solar panels on your roof, insulating your house better (to avoid heating your garden), lowering your thermostat in the winter and wearing a cardigan (as President Carter advocated, years ahead of his time), and increasing your thermostat in the summer to 78°F (believe me, it'll feel very comfortable if it is 95°F and humid outside) or forgoing air-conditioning altogether (there is a movement for that, too, if you are interested). These actions are directly related to our relationship with Nature.

You can also explore any of the movements in this chapter, via the web or books listed in the Appendix, although a direct interaction with Nature is ultimately more meaningful.

Lastly, meditating in Nature, or simply observing and appreciating its beauty on a walk through the woods, is very touching and helpful.

You may ask, "What does a deeper connection to my cat or a begonia have to do with solving our environmental problems?" Let me answer by saying that any place is a good place to begin connecting with Nature in a deeper, more aware, and more conscious way, since the effect is cumulative. The deeper you connect in one area, the more the effect spreads into adjacent areas (I know from experience). The more you realize your interconnectedness with Nature on all levels, the more you are likely to become interested in more serious environmental matters, like hydraulic fracturing, strip mining, waste disposal and recycling, or acid rain. As a matter of fact, baby steps are the perfect way to start.

Chapter 5

HEALTHY SOIL = HEALTHY ENVIRONMENT = HEALTHY BODY

"The nation that destroys its soil, destroys itself."

—*Franklin Delano Roosevelt*
(1882-1945)

"The soil is the great connector of lives, the source and destination of all. It is the healer and restorer and resurrector, by which disease passes into health, age into youth, death into life. Without proper care for it we can have no community, because without proper care for it we can have no life."

—*Wendell Berry*
(1934-)

EEP LIVING INVOLVES A DEEPER AWARENESS OF, and involvement with, everything in our everyday life, and so it does when it comes to growing food, the most fundamental of all human activities. Rudolph Steiner said something long ago that may not be obvious until we consider it deeply. In Lecture One of his Agriculture Course, he declared that "agriculture. . .alone makes possible the physical life of Man on Earth." Indeed, the development of human civilization, and the emergence of culture, did not begin until the advent of agriculture about ten thousand or so years ago. Before that time, smatterings of nomadic hunter-gatherer hordes roamed the Earth in search of roots, berries, nuts and seeds, edible greens and an occasional paleo roast.

Perhaps you have seen the bumper sticker *No Farms, No Food*. It implies *No Agriculture, No Civilization*. The word culture, which we relate to the arts and a more refined way of living, actually comes from the Latin cultus, "to tend," and from the French colere, "to till," while ager is Latin for "field." Therefore agri-culture means tilling the field, which shows just how symbiotic and entwined the relationship between agriculture and culture is. Agriculture assures our existence and is a prerequisite for culture, since we are unable to move up Maslow's hierarchy of needs without a steady and assured supply of nourishing food.

Agriculture deals with our human manipulation of the God-given soil and land we have been handed, and we have the power to do responsible as well as irresponsible things with it. Good agriculture assures a good existence. You might ask what bad agriculture is. The answer to that has played itself out in the Western world since the mid-nineteenth century, but has become much more acute in the past sixty or so years. Let me briefly frame the flaws in the system that currently produces most of the Western food supply, which will make it clear why it's high time for an agricultural paradigm shift; and, more importantly, I will showcase already existing trends and alternatives that point in the direction of possible and better agricultural futures.

A bit of history

In sedentary agricultural societies, crops are grown in the same area year after year, and soils become prone to depletion, while nomadic cultures live a sustainable life because they move on when they have eaten everything in a particular territory and the soil can then regenerate. But a nomadic way of life only works for small groups of people, while agriculture creates a basis for population growth and the forming of culture. While much of the developing world still gets a lot of its food from small "organic" subsistence farming plots, the West has shown the world what happens when both plot scale and output grow exponentially with the help of heavy-duty machinery. Large farms in the 1800s might have had a hundred-plus acres; a large farm today covers upwards of two thousand, and up to tens of thousands of acres.

Soil depletion was first noticed in the early 1800s, and the response was the new husbandry system of mixed farms. This system intensified yields by fertilizing crops with manure to avoid the practice of letting a portion of land lie fallow to self-regenerate over a period of time. Large-scale industrialized conventional farming, which is based on high energy input, began in earnest after World War II and was the result of both the Industrial Revolution of the mid-nineteenth century and the Green Revolution of the 1950s. Originally the goal of the latter was to feed masses of people cheaply, but it also resulted in the astonishing worldwide population explosion of the twentieth century. The increase in scale of this type of farming can be mind-boggling. Have you ever driven across the flat mid-West and beheld the enormous stretches of corn and wheat fields as far as the eye can see and then some, or a California almond orchard with rows and rows of trees that don't seem to end? You might have scratched your head at the logistics of taking care of such vast expanses. Impossible without huge machinery and lots of fuel, which made these enormous monocultures possible in the first place. How to get all those almond blossoms pollinated? How to tackle soil fertility on this scale? How to deal with pests and weeds? Old-fashioned tricks like crop rotation or spreading manure with a tractor are no longer practical. Pesticide-, fertilizer-, and fungicide-spraying crop dusters were the answer, chemicals raining down from the sky— remedies from without, not within.

What's wrong with big-ag?

Conventional big-ag, like our entire economy, is founded on the erroneous and recent belief that growth is everlasting. However, this system is unsustainable, not only because our planet is finite in size, but also because the cheapness of big-ag's crops, the efficiencies attained via monocultures, the ever-rising forced crop increases achieved with chemical pesticides and fertilizers, all have a price: ever poorer mineral deficient soil, soil erosion (as much as two billion tons each year in the U.S.), an alarming reduction in biodiversity (weeds, insects, birds, and animals all need more diverse ecosystems than those produced exclusively by wheat or corn for thousands of acres on end), insect and bird reduction as a result of pesticide contamination and monocultured crops, ground water contamination due to pesticide and fertilizer runoff (the fish get sick from the water, and so do we), one-size-fits-all crops and techniques regardless of local conditions and ecology, the farmer's loss of connection to his local ecosystem, and the *pesticide treadmill*, which is another name for chemical pesticide dependency. While the system created big short-term results with enormous crop increases and the population explosion of the twentieth century, we are increasingly recognizing the problems this chemical dependency has created. In this system, "each crop is grown in isolation and individual issues such as nutrition, pests and diseases are all addressed individually rather than as part of the whole system," Paul Kristiansen and Charles Merfield point out in *Organic Agriculture*. See the relationship here as well to the way we heal our body parts separately. This agricultural model fulfilled the desire for the highest yield at the lowest cost by striving to be as efficient mechanically, and as technologically advanced, as possible by addressing the challenges of pests and weeds with poisons. But it has become evident in recent years that chemical pesticides and synthetic fertilizers have not been the best solution for a number of reasons. The list of detrimental consequences from this type of farming is long, from chemical run-offs into the ground water, to pesticide resistance after the passage of a few years, farm workers' exposure to poisons, insect and bird die-offs (e.g., bee colony collapse syndrome due to neonicotinoid use), loss of biodiversity due to crop monocultures, cross pollination of GMO crops with neighboring non-GMO crops, consumers' ingestion of poison residues, depletion of the soil from being enriched artificially, and destabilization of the natural ecological balance in general.

Another consideration is that pesticides, herbicides, and synthetic fertilizers are costly to manufacture, expensive to buy, and their prices keep going up with rising energy costs. Between increasing costs for these products, potentially diminishing returns, and increasing environmental and health problems associated with conventional farming, our current big-ag system has become a recipe for disaster and a huge liability. Due to our underlying cultural values, we have created a profitable system that produces a lot of food. It is not, however, a system that is designed around growing the most nutritious, healthy and best tasting food while maintaining a balanced ecosystem. The food that comes from the current system has been cultivated to transport well (tomatoes with tough outer skins, and cubic watermelons—no joke, although they didn't last), to look good (taste comes second—this makes for watery tomatoes and strawberries), and to have uniform shapes (so they can be neatly packed and neatly stacked).

We are now learning the hard way that the single-minded focus on profitability ultimately exploits and depletes the soil and the environment at the expense of our health and our future. Laments farmer author Keith Stewart, in *Its a Long Road to a Tomato*, "We get cheap food, yes, but we pay for it later."

Agriculture stands at the intersection of Man and Nature. Yet we have increasingly adopted a singularly human-centric, strong-handed, and enemy-oriented way to work with Nature to produce food—kill the pests, kill the weeds, douse the soil with fertilizer if it doesn't want to produce more, tweak the plant genes and splice some desirable features into them to make them behave exactly how we want them to behave. Along the way, we have lost the co-operative relationship with Nature, resulting in detachment from it, together with a loss of sustainability. We have attempted to make up the system's perceived shortcomings with technology. But these corrective measures are turning out to be unsustainable, unhealthy, and fickle short-term solutions.

Ecological resilience, on the other hand, is an indicator of how permanent a system is in and of itself. Biodynamic farmer, professor, and author Fred Kirschenmann emphasizes that our conventional monocultured agriculture has thrived over the past sixty years because we have experienced an unusual period of relatively stable weather patterns. We cannot, however, as we are beginning to discover, rely on this in the long run. Kirschenmann also warns that our water tables have sunk to half 1960 levels, which means that plants have to be more drought resistant in the future. And biodiversity is crucial as it adds to the stability of an ecosystem. Monocultures have to be propped up with ever more fertilizer and pesticide/herbicide brews to keep producing, and they are prone to collapse under stressful conditions like extended drought or rainfall.

Instead, we must create more resilient agro-ecosystems in the future, polycultures that promote diversity. What has happened to our soil and the environment in general as a consequence of big-ag practices, to farm workers' health, and to our own health over the past century and a half is not making industrial agriculture look so good any longer.

While I could go on and on, this chapter is not meant to be a critique of conventional agriculture, although becoming aware of what we do *not* want serves as the basis for creating what we *do* want. I believe that we will come to see the present Western agricultural system historically as a short-term transitional solution that helped us to redefine our agricultural values and priorities in preparation for a shift to better models. Let's leave this outline of our existing conundrum behind and turn to the exciting developments in agriculture to frame alternative and possibly even better ways to grow food than the original organic way of the nineteenth century, negate the argument that only big-ag and GMOs can conquer world hunger, and provide you with ammunition for navigating your own food supply sources.

What now?

If you have only jumped on the farming and food bandwagon recently, your head may be spinning at the proliferation of terms relating to how we grow food these days. What is better for my family, locally or organically grown food? What is *fair trade?* What on Earth is *biodynamic farming?* Why should I join a *CSA?* What's so controversial about GMOs?

My coffee source sells bird-friendly and shade-grown coffee; what the heck is that? What is *permaculture?* How about the depletion of the oceans through overfishing? What about egg standards and the meat industry? Grass-fed versus corn-fed meat; free-range, cage-free, or battery-raised chickens for eggs; wild caught versus farm-raised fish; pasteurized and homogenized versus raw dairy products? It can be overwhelming when all you are trying to do is cook a healthy meal for your family. Yet such are our times and choices. With increasing awareness of all things agricultural, we create more variations and in turn get more choices. While agriculture encompasses all foods we grow, animal and vegetable, the focus here is on plant-based foods and the relationship between healthy soil and healthy body. I will discuss the meat quandary in the next chapter, on our relationship with food.

Some general thoughts about new agricultural models before looking at specifics. A very important aspect is their long-term perspective and idea of stewardship of the land to preserve it for future generations, something that indigenous cultures have always done, but that we have forgotten and need to relearn. New models are about replenishing the soil, putting minerals back into it that we have taken out, and preventing erosion. They are about *preserving the principal.* If you used up your retirement capital instead of living off the interest, you would run out of money soon.

Many new agricultural models go beyond the singular purpose of growing food for profit. They incorporate knowledge of local conditions, social responsibility, and paying fair wages certified through the fair-trade label. These are models whose intent it is to create win-win situations by maintaining healthy soil, a healthy ecosystem, promoting the health of those who eat what comes from it, as well as those who work the farms. New agricultural models are co-creative, which means that they work *with* Nature, not against it, in navigating pests, diseases, or more erratic weather patterns. But their foremost priority may be to grow the most nutritious and healthy foods for us.

Big-time idealism? If we can imagine it, we can create it, and the models are already out there. Yet a farm is a business if it is to sell its products. All sorts of hybrid systems between the two extremes have sprung up. They may be compromises, but their output is still healthier than that of the humongous monocultured industrial farms, and they are attempts at improving things, a step in the right direction.

Healthy soil

We must begin with a thought on soil, the basis for all agriculture. Healthy, fertile soil looks like Mississippi Mud Pie with critters—crumbly, almost black, richly moist, loose and soft, with creepy crawlies in it, the more the merrier.

Such rich soil is the result of an ongoing interaction among decaying organic matter, manure and compost, the critters that aerate it, and plant roots. Fertile soil is rich in minerals and trace elements, which the roots pull up for their growth and proliferation and which end up in the produce we eat. Not only are plants grown in mineral-rich soil strong, vigorous, and healthy, as well as more disease and weather resistant, they are also much more nourishing. We need less of such nutritious foods, while foods grown in poor soil leave us yearning for more.

Organics

Organic is the most widely recognized term for a less poisonous way of farming. It is not the end-all and necessarily best way to grow food, but it's a good start, and since most people are familiar with the term, we may as well begin here before expanding into what else is out there. In broad strokes, the main principle of organic agriculture is to refrain from using chemical fertilizers and pesticides. That sounds simple enough, but is not once the scale increases and profit gets in the way, the big conundrum of our times. Usually labor and production efficiencies are achieved with increasing scale, at the same time as quality—usually—decreases, although farmer philosopher Fred Kirschenmann, for example, has been successfully farming a thirty-five-hundred-acre biodynamic farm for decades. The International Federation of Organic Agriculture Movement's (IFOAM), definition of *organic* is more encompassing than simply refraining from using chemicals, though, and stipulates, "A production system that sustains the health of soils, ecosystems and people. It relies on ecological processes, biodiversity and cycles adapted to local conditions, rather than the use of inputs with adverse effects. Organic agriculture combines tradition, innovation, and science to benefit the shared environment and promote fair relationships and a good quality of life for all involved." Yet Kristine Brandt and Jens Peter Mølgaard, of the Danish Institute of Agricultural Sciences, point out that "IFOAM standards do not spell out food quality as an aim of its production—so it is a byproduct."

In the past the most common methods of pest control were cultural—rotating crops and letting fields lie fallow, intercropping, maintenance of biodiversity on a farm, all methods that kept each species in balance within a farm's ecosystem and relied on specific and intimate local knowledge. With the rise of large-scale industrial agriculture, the introduction of large monocultured crops, and the loss of biodiversity and thus balance, as well as the ensuing loss of local knowledge, chemical pesticides and fertilizers were introduced as a one-size-fits-all counter-measure. The consequences of the use of such poisons—the pesticide treadmill, endangering farm workers' health, chemicals leaching into the groundwater, and ingesting pesticide residue-ridden produce—led to the development of biological control in organic and sustainable agriculture systems. Yet even biological control is just that, a control mechanism, reactionary and suppressive. Cornell University Professor of Entomology Ann Hajek explains that looking at pest management from a more ecological perspective, a "total system approach," or a sustainable approach, requires us to change totally how pest problems are viewed. Instead of asking how to control a specific pest, we would be asking why the pest *is* a pest. "This would entail understanding the 'weakness in the ecosystem' and why an organism has become a pest in the first place," she writes. "Like IPM (Integrated Pest Management), the goal would not be to eliminate the pest but to bring pest densities within acceptable limits," and this approach requires a thorough knowledge of the local ecosystem. Paul Kristiansen, of the University of New England in Australia, and Charles Merfield, of Lincoln University in New Zealand, thus conclude that the idea of pest control in an organic system "is the design and interaction of the farm as a whole that controls pests."

The many ways of organic

Organic farming, although developed in the early 1900s around the same time as another alternative farming movement, the biodynamic model, has only been heralded as a solution to many of the problems associated with conventional agriculture in recent decades. Until about a hundred and fifty years ago, all farming was "organic" because chemical fertilizers and pesticides did not exist. In the years since, the techniques of managing weeds, pests, and soil fertility organically on a larger scale have become quite complex and labor-intensive, and require an intricate knowledge of farming, the farm's biosystem, and the area's ecosystem, and organic farmers employ a combination of techniques to avoid using chemicals. Crop rotation ensures that different plants draw different nutrients from the soil over time and don't deplete it continuously of the same minerals. Pre-irrigation (removal of weeds before they go to seed to ensure the seeds cannot reproduce), soil solarization (trapping heat from the sun with help of a tarp to kill pests and weeds), burning, and flaming are all organic techniques, as is growing leguminous cover crops that are plowed under between regular plantings to add nutrients back to the soil. Other techniques include the use of specifically bred disease-resistant plant varieties, promoting a "habitat for beneficial insects, predatory birds, and mammals to minimize pests," use of naturally occurring chemicals and biological controls, and the mixed organic farm's reuse of its animal manure as fertilizer.

Several years ago, I saw vegetables labeled *organic* at Walmart and garlic from China labeled *organic* at my local supermarket. Huh? As it turns out, there are many different gradations of organic, from *organic* to "organic," from *shallow organic* to *deep organic*. John Ikerd, Professor Emeritus of Agriculture at the University of Missouri, laments, "Unfortunately, in efforts to increase productivity and profitability of organics, to make organic food more accessible to more people, organic agriculture is being transformed into industrial agriculture." Fred Kirschenmann and author Michael Pollan talk about the "organic compromise, because organic still operates within a profit-driven sociopolitical structure." Once organic agriculture shifted from principles of human health and sustainability to profitability and productivity, the definition became compromised. We might compare the compromises of *shallow organic* to an organic Twinkie, if there were such a thing. It would use organic ingredients, but the fundamental deep organic ideal of wholesome food is compromised because a Twinkie, organic or not, is not a wholesome food to begin with. Organic in its *deep* definition is a holistic agricultural system whose premises are to grow healthy, delicious, and nourishing food while maintaining healthy and rich soil as well as preserving the environment. *Shallow organic*, which is what the big-ag-org farms are doing, merely substitutes chemical inputs for acceptable inputs under the organic label. *Deep organic*, on the other hand, requires a total system change to a different paradigm, because it is value- and principle-based. John Ikerd says, "Early advocates of organic farming believed that human health was directly connected to the health of the soil." We are coming back full circle to this realization, and are beginning to understand that the sustainability issue is so much bigger than simply refraining from applying chemicals. As an interim conclusion, the organic label safeguards you at least from GMO products (more on those later), the worst chemicals, the most mineral poor produce, and assures a modicum of environmental concern.

Sustainable agriculture

You may already have heard the term *sustainable agriculture*. "Sustainable," according to the online Dictionary of Environment and Conservation, means "Capable of being sustained or continued over the long term, without adverse effects." The same dictionary defines "sustainable agriculture" as "an agricultural system that is ecologically sound, economically viable, and socially just. Sustainable agriculture uses techniques to grow crops and raise livestock that conserve soil and water, use organic fertilizers, practice biological control of pests, and minimize the use of non-renewable fossil fuel energy." Ikerd points out, "A sustainable agriculture must meet the needs of the present without compromising the opportunities of the future. A sustainable agriculture must be capable of sustaining an ever-renewing, regenerative, evolving, diverse, holistic, interdependent human society for as long as Earth receives energy from the Sun, the ultimate source of sustainability. . . . A sustainable agriculture is a permanent agriculture." It strives for a cyclical and thus long-term method that is based in a local ecosystem and remains viable indefinitely from a social and ecological perspective, with the emphasis on *indefinitely*. It is a permanent agriculture designed for the highest good of all, not Man alone, and is thus a co-operative effort between Man and Nature. Sustainable agriculture overlaps with deep organic and permaculture principles, which will become clear when I discuss permaculture. However, while *organic* and *biodynamic* certifications exist, there are no *sustainable* or *permaculture* certifications. *Sustainable* and *deep organic* agriculture are thus synonyms in their purest interpretation. If organic agriculture follows the industrial profit-driven model, on the other hand, it is not sustainable. Sustainable agriculture is a cyclical, self-contained, and permanent system, one that can go on eternally. At the risk of repeating myself, only a permanent system is truly sustainable, and such a system should not require biological control as a substitute for chemical pesticides in the long term. John Vandermeer, of the University of Michigan, makes this clear when he writes, "If it is the underlying structure of the system that is the problem in the first place, focusing on input substitution [biological control for chemical pest management, or organic fertilizer from outside the farm for chemical fertilizer] is putting a band-aid on a cancerous tumor."

Biodynamic farming

With biodynamic farming we are coming to a completely different agricultural principle. Biodynamic farming has been called über-organic or organic on steroids, because it goes way beyond the principles of organic and sustainable farming. It is philosopher Rudolph Steiner's brainchild and could also be called *holistic* or *spiritual* farming. Steiner equates a farm to a living entity, as the Gaia principle does the Earth. In Lecture Two of his Agriculture Course, Steiner explained that "a farm is true to its essential Nature...if it is conceived as a kind of individual entity in itself—a self-contained individuality." The Biodynamic Association defines "biodynamics" as a "holistic, ecological and ethical approach to farming, gardening, food and nutrition," while Demeter, the biodynamic certification organization, adds that biodynamics "note both the visible and invisible forces that create a healthy eco-system." This system goes above and beyond organic and sustainable agriculture because it considers, and works with, the influence of cosmic forces. Besides considering the farm as a living entity, biodynamic farmers work with planetary influences and aspects in determining the time for sowing and harvesting. Because biodynamic farmers understand just how crucial soil quality is, they also work with special biodynamic soil solutions throughout the season, which could be likened to homeopathic agricultural remedies. Because biodynamic farming works hand in hand with planetary influences on different plant parts, a gardening or farming calendar is issued for each year that specifies optimal gardening days for specific tasks such as planting greens or harvesting root vegetables.

Permaculture

Permaculture, like biodynamics, is another form of agriculture that goes above and beyond the principles of organics while sharing many values with sustainable farming. The term *permaculture* is a composite of the words *permanent* and *agriculture*, so a permanent culture *cum* agriculture. Each permaculture system is a custom application, entirely unique and modeled around specific local conditions such as weather and climate, indigenous plants, and local customs and circumstances. Industrial farming methods, in contrast, are not locale-specific but standardized, the way medical treatment methods are generally standardized. Vandermeer writes that "academic knowledge is general but shallow, whereas local knowledge is specific and deep. Many ecological processes are locality-specific, whereas industrial agriculture caused us to lose a lot of that local knowledge."

"In a well-designed [permaculture] system all or most of our needs are provided by outputs in the system, so that the system becomes a closed-energy cycle," Scottish author and permaculture expert Graham Bell writes. James Veteto, an assistant professor of anthropology at the University of North Texas, explains that "the overall aim of these design principles is to develop closed-loop, symbiotic, self-sustaining human habitats and production systems that do not result in ecological degradation or social injustice." The ideal permaculture farm is a closed-loop system that generates its own energy and reuses its own waste sustainably without degrading the environment. But the interpretation can go even beyond that, according to the Australian founder of permaculture, Bill Mollison: "Permaculture is the conscious design and maintenance of agriculturally productive ecosystems which have the diversity, stability, and resilience of natural ecosystems. It is the harmonious integration of landscape and people providing their food, energy, shelter and other material and non-material needs in a sustainable way."

In brief, permaculture strives to grow as large a variety of mostly perennial plants as possible, to provide food, fuel, fiber, medicine, and even construction material, explains Chuck Burr of the Permaculture Research Institute, on as compact a farm as possible, with minimal energy input, all the while working for the benefit of all of Nature and operating within a highly ethical system. In addition, the idea is to eliminate pollution, i.e., one-way waste output without further use in the system, true garbage.

Wow! These principles go way beyond growing food to also becoming socially and ecologically responsible, and growing plants for fiber and building materials. On this more encompassing scale, permaculture truly becomes a permanent or sustainable culture.

Mark Shepard, a permaculture instructor and farmer who practices permaculture in combination with biodynamics, stresses the deep symbiosis between culture and agriculture. He explains that, "without a truly sustainable agriculture, there would be no sustainable culture." He goes further still, into the history of agriculture and the history of civilization, and maintains that our agricultural model of the past ten thousand years has never been truly sustainable. He warns, "It has been the inherent unsustainability of the agriculture of the empire cultures that has helped them all to collapse periodically," intimating the same possibility exists for our own culture.

What do permaculture farms look like? They have been described as messy. Traditional agriculture grows crops horizontally in a single layer, in rows or fields, and usually, but not always, one crop per row, field, or bed. These traditional systems look organized to us because we have imposed our human sense of order on them. Traditional agriculture does not resemble Nature.

Permaculture systems, on the other hand, are deliberately designed, complex, and layered systems that emulate natural ecosystems and therefore do not conform to our human sense of order. That is why they look messy to us. Permaculture crops grow vertically on many different levels, the way plants grow in Nature. In Shepard's words, permaculture is a three-dimensional system when compared to traditional agriculture's one-dimensional or flat layout. Because permaculture farms always emulate the local ecosystem native to the farm's location, permaculture crops are native to the local ecosystem as well. While sustainable agriculture works within the context of a local ecosystem too, it grows many non-indigenous crops that have been introduced from other parts of the world, and that are not naturally adapted to the local ecosystem. This makes those plants potentially less resistant to pests, diseases, and more erratic weather patterns, while permaculture only grows indigenous plants where they are perfectly at home and well adapted. You would grow apples and chestnuts in a permaculture setting in the northeastern U.S. but not goji berries, which would grow just fine but are not native. Permaculture is more biodiverse than sustainable agriculture, because it grows a more complex combination of crops, and it does not fight weeds and wildflowers but works with them. This diversity of plants naturally promotes a proliferation of beneficial insects that minimize pests and diseases. The increased biodiversity makes the entire system more stable in the long term. Shepard states that, "as a general rule, the more diverse a system is, the more stable it is in the long term."

Another advantage of permaculture over sustainable agriculture entails more comprehensive rain absorption due to permaculture's three-dimensional design. While "row crops with their clean soil surface beneath them tend to allow rain to turn right off the fields," permaculture's many-layered verticalities of tree and shrub crops "slow the impact of the rainfall reducing the damage to soil structure," Shepard explains. Permaculture orchards require less or no fertilizer because the leaves and evergreen needles of its tree and shrub crops simply fall to the ground, where they decompose and become natural fertilizer. In addition, this leaf-and-needle layer protects the soil from erosion and water evaporation.

The last, and perhaps most important, permaculture characteristic is that many or all permaculture crops are perennial. This system works with fruit and nut trees and berry shrubs for a vertical layering of crops. To keep energy input on a permaculture farm to a strict minimum, sheep and geese may naturally manage grass, weeds, and wildflowers by feeding on them.

In conclusion, permaculture is more complex, more biodiverse, more stable, more resilient, more permanent, and thus more sustainable than sustainable agriculture. It is a new agricultural system modeled on the perennial crops available to hunter-gatherers before the advent of sedentary agriculture's annual grain and vegetable crops, while sustainable agriculture operates within the premises of the traditional agricultural model of the past ten thousand years, a model of horizontally spread-out annual crops that are not necessarily indigenous to the ecosystem they are grown in.

In Central America, a smaller version of a permaculture application, called a *milpa*, has been in use for millennia. A milpa is a planting system that emulates Nature, the way permaculture does, and incorporates a variety of environmentally but also nutritionally complementary crops, as Charles Mann explains in his best-seller *1491*. H. Garrison Wilkes, Professor Emeritus at the University of Massachussetts in Boston and a maize expert, calls the milpa "one of the most successful human inventions ever created." It's so sustainable that some of them have been cultivated for thousands of years. One such well-known nutritional grouping here in the Northeast is the Native American corn–bean–squash combination that has traditionally been cultivated as well as eaten together.

The sustainability of perennial crops

Since perennial crops play such a big role in permaculture, let's look at their advantages over annual crops. All our vegetables and grains are annual plants. The only perennial crops we currently cultivate widely are berry shrubs, as well as fruit and nut trees. Annual crops are very labor-intensive and costly, because new seeds are required each year, in addition to the labor involved in the endless tilling, planting, and plowing cycles. Because annual crops only have a few months to grow before being torn out or plowed under, their roots are shorter as well, and grow less deep than those of perennial crops. Thus, annuals are more prone to suffer during drought, in addition to which they draw up a lot fewer minerals than perennials with deeper and more extensive root systems. Moreover, the tilling and turning of the soil in the spring and fall, as well as soil exposure during the winter months, promote rapid topsoil erosion and quicker evaporation. Perennials are more resilient and more nutritious. Due to their deeper root systems, their mineral and protein content is up to one-third higher than that of annual crops. In addition, explains soil scientist Jerry Glover, "Their longer growing season and more extensive root systems make them more competitive against weeds and more effective at capturing nutrients and water." Perennial crops constitute a long-term investment. They are more economical than annual crops because they do not have to be laboriously re-sown every year, avoiding labor-intensive tilling and the annually reoccurring cost for new seeds, and minimizing or eliminating the need for fertilizer.

What about grains and seeds?

We are still missing a very important piece of the puzzle, the grain and seed crops. The world population has derived most of its staple foods and fibers from annual grains, seeds, and legumes ever since the advent of sedentary agriculture, as these provide a lot of quick and bundled energy. The bulk of our agricultural production consists of grains, oilseed, and legume crops, "occupying 75% of U.S. and 69% of global croplands," according to agricultural researchers Jerry Glover and John Reganold. While all of them are annual crops, there is a good reason why they have been favored. We selectively bred annuals for bigger yields and seed sizes, which gradually led away from the smaller-yield perennial grain and seed ancestors, and now dominate our food supply. Researchers are working on perennial versions of some grains and legumes, which is exciting because perennials are also more climate change resistant, in addition to offering the advantages presented above. This represents a crucial development in the history of agriculture. Research, development, and introduction of perennial seed and grain varieties, while running counter to the industrial-agricultural profit-based model, is the superior solution to arguing that world hunger can only be conquered with genetically modified crops.

Social models

In recent years social agricultural models have developed. One of them is Community Supported Agriculture (CSA). Between increasing awareness of the benefits of local food sources and the explosion of farmers markets in this country, it is likely that there are CSAs in your own backyard. A CSA is a farm that charges up front at the beginning of the growing season for the right to a share of its crops. In abundant years, this arrangement works to the customer's benefit; in lean years, the risk is spread among all CSA members.

There are working and non-working CSAs. Participating in a working CSA reduces the seasonal share cost. The seasonal shareholder helps to finance the purchase of seed and investment in labor and equipment through the up-front purchase of produce shares. As the concept has gained acceptance, there are now also egg and dairy, meat, and even flower CSAs.

On another social front, the fair-trade label assures that farm workers, here and abroad, are paid a living wage and not exploited. My food co-op has offered fair-trade bananas for years, and fair-trade coffee has become common.

OMG—GMOs

And now that I have written that ominous acronym, let's talk about GMOs, genetically modified organisms. While many countries already require labeling or have banned them outright, here in the U.S. we are still unwilling guinea pigs in a government-sponsored experiment, because we don't yet have GMO labeling in place. Unless you buy organic, you don't know whether you are eating GMOs or not, although it is known that most corn and soy crops are genetically altered. Produce now employs a labeling system that identifies organic produce (a five-number PLU code starting with a "9," such as 94011 for an organic non-GMO banana), GMO produce (a five-number PLU code starting with an "8," such as 84011 for a GMO banana), and conventionally grown produce (a four-number PLU code, such as 4011 for a conventionally grown banana). Check it out in the produce section at your local supermarket. However, GMO products do not have to be identified on packaged food, nor do fish or meat. Torr points out that "approval for commercial release of transgenic crops is based on scientific information provided voluntarily by companies producing genetically engineered crops," a practice that goes against scientific procedures for third-party verification and is of concern, to say the least.

What, exactly, *are* genetically modified organisms? Genetic modification alters the genetic material of a plant or an animal by splicing in desirable traits from another species. GMO Awareness points out, in the definition on its website, that "genetic engineering forcefully breaches the naturally-occurring barriers between species." We are forcing our will on Nature without knowing and understanding the long-term consequences. Scientists, however, have either already discovered, or are predicting, serious and troublesome consequences of the use of genetically engineered crops, whether through ingestion, introduction into Nature, or in the underlying, strictly profit-driven motives of the large biotechnical corporations that are behind the technology. Molecular geneticist Ricarda Steinbrecher confirms that GMO crops can interbreed with non-GMO species. The scary thing is, as Dr. Steinbrecher cautions, the "completely unpredictable" side effects of GMO crops, such as "genetically modified salmon reared in Scotland that was engineered to grow fast, but which also unpredictably turned green." Steinbrecher warns that the genes of modified organisms are unstable in later generations, resulting in these kinds of unknown consequences. Another danger of GMO crops is that the plants weaken due to genetic forcing of characteristics external to their own makeup. This stresses the plant and makes it unfit in the long term, Steinbrecher points out. On a different note, an ethical concern is that the large biochemical companies may not necessarily act out of humanitarian motives, but instead seem purely profit-driven, with the single goal of monopolizing the rights to the genes, their manufacture, and their distribution, in addition to the herbicide and pesticide business they already control.

Conclusion

Evolution is about shifting and growing while keeping worthwhile knowledge and wisdom previously acquired and shedding what does not work and becomes obsolete. In that way Nature—and we are a part of it—becomes ever more complex and diversified. What you can personally take away from the information presented in this chapter is that the source of your food is incredibly important, and that the parameters of how we as a culture grow our food are changing. No wonder the consumption of organics has flourished so incredibly in recent decades. Healthy soil is tantamount to healthy food, because it assures that your food is mineral rich and nutritious, which in turn assures you a healthy body that gets its nutrients from the soil as opposed to pills. The importance of perennial crops should not be overlooked either—not only because they are more mineral- and protein-rich than annual foods due to their deeper and extensive root systems, but also because they are more resilient in face of more erratic weather patterns. In that regard, John Vandermeer stresses the importance of recognizing, not only how traditional systems solve problems, but how they avoid them in the first place. This is what positive-oriented holistic approaches do. In healthcare, for example, we will hopefully shift to becoming wellness- instead of illness-oriented, and in agriculture I hope we become wellness- instead of profit-oriented as well, both spiritually connected proactive approaches from within. The question is what value system we subscribe to. We have had to learn the hard way, paying with illness and a polluted environment, that a profit- and growth-driven agriculture produces win–lose scenarios, while a sustainable agriculture produces win–win scenarios. Finding ways out of a crisis always requires creativity and lateral thinking. Straight-laced organics is only the tip of finding new ways to grow food and where agriculture might be headed in the next decades. Ultimately, it's not about coming up with *the* best agricultural system, because each local condition mandates a custom solution.

The more aware you become personally, the more invested you become in researching the sources of what you put on your family table, and the more relevant questions you ask your local farmers, the stronger the movement towards sustainable forms of agriculture grows. Because the Hudson Valley, where I live, grows so much food for the entire New York Metropolitan Area and is so food-oriented, interest in farming has grown tremendously, and there are exciting new developments on the horizon. A new community-cum-farming initiative recently formed around the five-farmer organic Chester Agricultural Center and the adjacent Green Onion farmer's market, whose vision correlates with the original meaning of agriculture—culture that arises from farming. This local initiative brings together farming, a farmer's market, food offerings, and culture in various forms from music, to poetry readings, to talks, to movies—one of the many avenues to our agricultural future.

How to connect more deeply with how your food is grown

Farmer's markets and farm stands have sprouted up just about everywhere, and farmers like to connect with their customers and get to know them. Start a relationship with the places you buy your food from. Ask your local farmers how they deal with pests and soil fertility. Ask whether or not they use GMO seeds. Ask about their difficulties in dealing with unpredictable weather patterns. I know several local farmers, our local French pâtisserie owners, and the owners of some of the farm-to-table restaurants in my town. It's so much more fun to buy from people I know and can have a chat with, and who care deeply about food, than to go to the supermarket.

The higher price of organics is a big hurdle for many (although considering you buy better health for yourself and the environment, it's also a worthwhile up-front investment and offers the hope of a reduction in medical problems down the road). I buy organics in bulk from a food co-op instead of the local supermarket. That way I get more variety and a better price, and I share the cases and crates with friends (and a lot of networking gets done at the monthly co-op deliveries, too).

Consider shifting budget priorities away from clothing, electronics, or high-priced event tickets to higher quality foods, which is what we have done.

Join a working or non-working CSA if you live in the country; in exchange for a few hours of work each week, the share price drops.

Since you vote with your food dollars, the more sustainably grown produce you buy, the bigger the movement gets, and the more the word gets out that that's what people want. It's the way to personally vote for health and against poison.

While this chapter is about plant based food, the natural extension of buying produce from your local farmers is to buy eggs, honey, dairy, and meat locally as well. Not only will you gain a closer connection to your food sources, you will also strengthen your local economy instead of the big corporation that runs the supermarket.

Buy, cook, and eat more plant-based foods, period.

Chapter 6

FOOD TO NOURISH, NOT FOOD AS FUEL

"Food probably has a very great influence on the condition of men. Wine exercises a more visible influence, food does it more slowly but perhaps just as surely. Who knows if a well-prepared soup was not responsible for the pneumatic pump or a poor one for a war?"

—*Georg Christoph Lichtenberg (1742–1799)*

Introduction

DEEP LIVING ENTAILS A DEEPER awareness of, and involvement with, everything that pertains to our everyday life, and so it does when it comes to what we put into our body, the food and beverages we eat and drink to nourish ourselves as a basis for our existence. These days feeding your family can be a complex, very involved, and potentially frustrating endeavor if you begin to dig deeper into food matters. A while ago, after I had labored over a tedious-to-make homemade version of a famous Italian chocolate hazelnut spread, which involved soaking hazelnuts for several hours and melting cocoa butter over a low flame, my then fourteen-year-old son tasted the result, rolled his eyes, and said "Can't you just buy the real stuff?" And when my then ten-year-old daughter asked whether we could have pizza on Friday night, and I replied, "Sure, I can make pizza on Friday night," she, too, rolled her eyes in despair and replied, "No, I mean, can we *buy* it?"

What is it with food these days? Everybody seems to have the definite answer about *what* to eat or what *not* to eat, which diet to lose weight on, or that we all need to become vegetarians or vegans to save the world or avoid getting cancer, or which supplements ensure better memory (gingko biloba?) or a longer life (resveratrol?). In addition, especially in America, there seems to be a belief that *bad-for-you* foods taste good but make you overweight and sick, and that *good-for-you* foods taste bad but promote wellness (those beliefs are less prevalent in traditional food cultures like France or Italy, where they do enjoy their butter, cream, meat, or olive-oil-drenched vegetables with a lot less guilt than we do on this side of the Atlantic). Here, we have developed a controversial relationship with food. My fellow graduate Heidi Feichtinger agrees. She writes, "In America, we believe healthy eating involves suffering; after all, delicious food and dessert are simply sinful!" (Doesn't that ring a religious bell?) No wonder such thinking contributes to food-related disorders like bulimia and anorexia. As Feichtinger says, "So many people see food as the enemy."

I have come to see food as my ally in building and maintaining an energetic and strong body, food that not only sustains me but also nourishes my soul, food as celebration, food as an opportunity to spend time with family and friends. If you have not yet made peace with food, this chapter will provide you with food for thought (pun intended) to inspire a shift from the shallower perspective of food as fuel to a deeper and more meaningful view of embracing food as nourishment for body and soul, and enjoying all the experiences that go with it—food shopping or even growing it, caring about where your food comes from and how it was grown, the meditative joys of food preparation, the convivial satisfaction of feasting with family and friends, and the meaningfulness of connecting with cultural or ethnic food traditions. These are all elements that have only been embraced by the exploding American food culture fairly recently.

The Strawberry Quandary and the Quality of Food

A clamshell of tasteless strawberries from California costs about two dollars on sale at my supermarket, while locally grown strawberries easily go for more than double that when they are finally available in June. The small and deeply red local ones taste the way strawberries *should* taste—sweet, sun ripened, intense, and with that distinct strawberry flavor.

In Part One, I spoke about how we express our personal values and priorities. One way to express value is through how much money we are willing to spend on certain things. We have been trained by big-ag and the government to expect our food to be cheap. Michael Pollan, author of *In Defense of Food*, reports that food spending went down from 17.5 percent of income in 1960 to 9.9 percent today. But why? Once you appreciate the intimate relationship between food and well-being, the question pops up: Why *not* spend good money for good food?

Usually, the food we get so cheaply is qualitatively not worth as much as the food that costs more, an aspect science sweeps under the rug in this case because it serves the profit-driven cause of the food industry, and not the consumer's health or quality of life. While the food industry keeps harping on the fact that organic food doesn't taste different from conventional food, or that its nutritional content is not much different, it neglects to mention that corn- and antibiotic-fed feedlot beef, for example, is downright unhealthy for your body (besides the fact that it sickens the animals and harms the environment), while grass-fed beef is much more wholesome; or that organically grown produce and grains have more minerals and nutrients because they were grown in richer, healthier soil, while conventionally grown plant based foods have pesticide residue, in addition to contributing to environmental pollution.

Ripeness, flavor, smell, aroma, and other qualitative food characteristics, such as its energetic aspect, cannot be measured in the same way as calories and nutrient percentages. Yet we all clearly prefer a strawberry that tastes like a strawberry should taste to those large, watery, and spongy half-white-half-red things in plastic clamshells, once we have become aware of the difference between the two.

Food is what builds and maintains the body and contributes in a major way to our health. Herbert Koepf, of the Fields Agricultural Institute in East Troy, Wisconsin, writes, "The final measure of nutritional quality lies in the organism which consumes the food." They used to say, about computers, "garbage in, garbage out." The same goes for the relationship between food and body. Within a few weeks of switching our two cats to a homemade raw meat diet a while ago, their vitality increased noticeably, their coats turned shiny and shimmering, and our older cat's body self-regulated back to an ideal weight. *The better the food quality, the better your health.*

Produce grown on a small local farm without pesticides and chemical fertilizers, and picked at the height of ripeness, or artisanal sausages and cheeses made with passion in small batches, are precious. Why on Earth should the price of such foods not reflect the difference between them and the supermarket alternative? In France people would rather drive a banged-up car than forgo oysters and champagne for Christmas. Quality food is a true priority for the French. I am well aware that we all have to juggle monthly food budgets—I do, too. But we are also in control of the household budget and *how* we spend our money. You *can* choose to spend more on food and less on something else (brand-name jeans and purses, cable TV and cellphone services, big cars, or poorly insulated homes are just some things that come to mind). *How* you spend your dollars is an expression of your values and priorities. Consumers often get misled by the question "Does it taste different?" when trying to understand whether to pay a higher price for organic food. The question should be different: How do you *feel*, how *well* are you? It has been established that organic food is much more mineral and vitamin rich than conventional food (our soils are depleted, though organic soil is a bit better) and does not contain toxic pesticide residues the way conventional produce does, besides protecting the environment and the farm hands' health. If that is not enough incentive, I don't know what is.

The price of food should rightfully reflect the labor, love, time, and environmental circumstances that went into growing or preparing it and providing its inherent quality. We ought to pay for this difference in quality without argument because it contributes in a major way to our health and wellbeing.

Nutritionism, the Western Diet, and some current food beliefs

When my husband comes home from work, he usually heads to the refrigerator in the hope of finding a quick pre-dinner snack, and he often exclaims in frustration, "There's no *food*. What can I eat?" That is of course not true. There is cheese, there is fruit, there are vegetables, there are milk, wine, and seltzer, there is bread, there are eggs and butter, and various condiments, nut butters, and such.

What he means is that there is no ready-to-eat packaged snack food.

How, then, did we end up with ready-to-eat, factory-made foods that come in packages? How did we end up disassembling foods into their nutritional components or nutrients? How did we get to believe we could do better than Nature by manufacturing foods that contain only supposedly beneficial nutrients? Where does the belief come from that we can only feed the growing world population if we manufacture food in factories, create GMO crops, grow animals for meat on feed lots, and spray fruits and vegetables with chemical pesticides, and the soil with synthetic fertilizers? Who decided that food had to be cheap, and why? Who decided that we had no time to cook from scratch, and why? Whose values and priorities *are* they?

The last big change to our diet began with industrialization in the nineteenth century, which entailed a shift to a culture based on high energy input. Already then, the soil quality began to suffer from mineral depletion, which resulted in less nutritious foods. The nail in the coffin for our diet, though, was The Green Revolution of the 1940s, which was marketed as a method to feed the millions cheaply or save them from starvation. In reality, its government policies fed profit-oriented agri-businesses at the expense of public health. This last food revolution is the real culprit in the dramatic rise in cancer, diabetes, obesity, and heart disease in all Westernized cultures. The Green Revolution's Western Diet is cheap, nutrient-deficient, and based on engineered profit-generating food products made in factories. This shift towards engineered food products went hand in hand with a shift in various food-related beliefs.

Here's an example of how food becomes an industry. If I make an omelet with eggs, vegetables, and herbs from the garden, the ingredient list is simple and the supply line direct (that is, if I get the eggs from my own chickens or the local farmer). It is still pretty simple if I buy the eggs and vegetables at a supermarket.

If, on the other hand, I buy Western omelet mix in a carton at the supermarket, I am supporting the Western omelet-mix factory, the big-ag egg supplier, the big-ag pork business (for the bits of ham), and the big-ag vegetable grower (for the bits of peppers), whose products all have to be transported at a cost to the Western omelet-mix factory. I am also supporting the omelet-mix carton maker, the supermarket that sells the mix, and probably some chemical company that makes food preservatives and food coloring. In short, I am supporting The Economy.

Earlier, I wrote about the Erector-set mentality that attempts unsuccessfully to understand the whole as the sum of its parts, whether we are talking about bodies, food, soil, or anything else that is natural. Since we have come to believe in ultimate scientific truths, we currently believe in ultimate and best treatments for medical conditions, as we believe in ultimate and best diets based on scientific formulas—powdered infant formula is perhaps the ultimate aberration. But it is a mistake to believe that the food industry will cure our ills with miracle foods. Instead, the marriage of government policies with the profit-driven food industry's deceitful approach has produced "the one diet that reliably makes. . . people sick," as Michael Pollan puts it. Gyorgy Scrinis's term for the misguided science behind it is "nutritionism."

As a matter of fact, it's just been revealed that a Harvard research team was paid off by the sugar industry in the 1960s to divert attention from sugar, as one of the culprits of heart disease (and, as we now know, of many more afflictions), to fat. This deception lies at the root of our fat fear and of an entire industry that manufactured low- and no-fat products. It made an entire culture sicker.

The good-food–bad-food syndrome is another myth. For a while eggs were considered *bad*, because we believed cholesterol was bad, and egg white omelets became the "healthy" thing to eat. Fat became the other big bad food, as mentioned above, and the food industry made low-fat and non-fat versions of milk, cheese, yogurt, butter! (*I Can't Believe It's Not Butter* is the name of an actual product), bacon (the turkey version), creating a large demand (and big business) for manufactured food products that are far removed from Nature (just read a butter substitute ingredient label to understand *how* far removed from Nature). This approach is not objective but pseudo-scientific, because it is slanted for the specific purpose of creating a need where none existed previously, for financial gain. Of course, we never quite understood how the French could eat butter and cream in supposedly sinful quantities without incurring increased rates of heart disease and high cholesterol. We called it the *French paradox* because the objective science behind it was not truthfully disclosed (the truth is that we *need* fat in our diet). *We have believed in the imperfection of Nature instead of the imperfection of our culture.*

That is what beliefs can do. Yet an omelet (made with yolks *and* whites), some herbs, some leftover vegetables, and served with a salad, is a wholesome dinner you can make from scratch in minutes, almost as fast as using Western omelet mix (just don't eat three eggs with bacon for breakfast every day—it's all about balance and diversity).

Other food myths include the idea that we need lots of dairy to get our calcium (a marketing ploy by the dairy industry, as milk-intolerant Asians live healthily without dairy because they get their calcium from greens), that more protein is better (a ploy by the meat industry), that white rice and white bread without a crust (i.e., Wonderbread) are more sophisticated than whole grain versions (this myth is very old; white flour was the *ne plus ultra* in olden times simply because it was more expensive to make than the whole grain kind), and that fats that are solid at room temperature are bad (coconut oil, for example, is not, nor is butter from grass-fed cows; what is really bad are the solid manufactured hydrogenated fats such as shortening). For a complete discussion of all this misinformation, and much, much more, see Sally Fallon and Mary Enig's *Nourishing Traditions*.

In conclusion, if you eat the foods Nature made, you can ignore the tedious food labels.

Food energetics

In the quantum universe, everything is energy. The New Physics has turned our understanding of matter, and of the universe, upside down and inside out. In the broadest of strokes, the theory says that everything in the universe is made of energy, and that solid matter only *appears* solid to our limited five senses but is not so in reality. In keeping with this line of thinking, the intake of food is an intake of energy. Energy has different frequencies, and different frequencies have different qualities. You can feel the presence of a person or an animal in a room, even if you don't see her. You perceive her energy. When you feel good in someone's presence, or you meet someone whom you don't feel comfortable with, you pick up on her energetic quality. If you compare a lettuce that has been sitting in a supermarket bin for a few days to one picked fresh this morning, you might perceive an energetic difference between the two, finding the fresh picked lettuce, say, more vibrant. This means that different kinds of foods have different energetic qualities, which in turn may influence our body in different ways. Transference and absorption of positive energy is the reason behind blessing food before a meal, a connection the Japanese researcher Masaru Emoto made in his famous water experiments, in which he infused water with love simply by pronouncing the word. Processed foods, made in a factory from ingredients we can barely pronounce, do not have life energy. They are dead foods, because their origin is so far removed from Nature. The closer to Nature a food is, the more life energy it has. Your rational mind may try to tell you that food is food (the food industry tries to, anyway), wherever it comes from. But ask your heart the dif-

ference between an Oreo cookie and a sun-ripened tomato from
your garden, and you'll grasp it immediately.

The quality of a food, or a food's characteristics, according to
nutrition counselor Steve Gagné, is embedded in it through the
manner in which the food was created—whether, for example, it
grew slowly or fast; down into the ground or up into the air; was
processed or not and how much, or came directly from Nature to
table; how an animal, whose meat we eat, lived, what it ate, how it
was treated, and how it was slaughtered. We incorporate each
food's energy into our own system when we eat it, he explains.
Rudolf Steiner noted over a hundred years ago that the lack of quality and life energy in our food has already implications on our overall state of being. He argued even then, that long ago, that food
had lost its spiritual properties to nourish the brain and the will,
and that our will power was therefore compromised (maybe there
is a grain of truth in this—think of all the people who unsuccessfully try to quit smoking or losing weight although they have good
intentions).

Physician, author, and nutrition counselor Otto Wolff explains
that plant food is more energetic than animal food because it produces energy directly from sunlight, and that raw plant food is yet
more energetic than cooked plant food. He notes that most animals
we consume eat plant food (except for some seafood, we actually do
not eat meat-eating animals and birds of prey, although some indigenous people do on occasion, and there may well be an energetic
reason behind it), and are thus once removed from sun energy, while
predators are twice removed from sun energy. Wolff considers meat
a stimulant, which is precisely the reason for its disproportionate
rise in the Western diet. As such, the rise in meat consumption is

DEEP LIVING

literally an addiction. To put this into perspective, consider that Germans ate about forty pounds of meat annually per person in 1850, while Americans consumed 138 pounds of meat per person in the 1950s, which rose to a shocking 270 pounds per person per year in 2012, more than any other place in the world. No wonder there are so many advocates for vegetarian and vegan diets. The staggering increase in meat consumption, coupled with the population explosion and toxic industrialized meat production methods and fish farming practices, have had disastrous environmental effects. But Wolff is no proponent of a vegan diet or of a raw food diet, since he believes that vegans, who consume no animal products whatsoever, not even honey or eggs, tend to become "remote from life" or "unable to deal with life" due to the lack of meat energy in their diet. With meat it is quality, not quantity, something New York University nutrition professor and author Marion Nestlé agrees with, advocating that we reduce our meat consumption to "condiment" quantities.

In regard to food energy, a more esoteric consideration is Steiner's argument for eating more perennial plants than we currently do. He argues that perennial plants have a fundamentally different energy due to their deeper and more expansive root systems, which, he maintains, allows them to absorb outer planet forces that are transferred to our nervous systems when we consume those plant foods. He says that annual plants, on the other hand, reinforce the inner planet aspects of reproduction and hyper-reproductive growth (his explanation for the world population explosion) and lack the necessary strength for manifesting the spirit in the physical. Regardless of what we make of this latter argument, crop scientists Kevin Murphy and Lori Hoagland have shown that perennial grains actually do have a higher protein and mineral content than our annual versions. For that reason, and for reasons of sustainability (annuals require a much higher energy input), "breeders have begun to develop perennial versions of wheat, sorghum, sunflowers and legumes," Glover and Reganold note, a promising development we have already discussed in the chapter on agriculture. *The inherent quality of the foods we eat directly translates into our level of energy and well-being.*

In summary, whether you're interested in the more esoteric interpretations of food energetics or not, it does make intuitive sense that fresh local foods would have more life energy than processed foods from a factory or produce that has travelled long distances on a truck and then sat in a supermarket produce bin for days. If you are still doubtful of the relevance of food energetics, watch Morgan Spurlock's documentary *Super Size Me.* I am convinced he not only became ill because of the *quantities* of fast food he consumed, but also because of its low energetic quality.

Slow Food or the Celebration of Food

My children enjoy the fun foods my husband buys when he is out and about with them when they run errands, yet they both acknowledge that one of the best things in life is escargots, the French snails with hot garlic butter and warm crusty baguette we sometimes have for a special family dinner. Fun foods have dozens of ingredients, many of which we can barely pronounce, while snails come with a simple garlic–parsley–shallot butter, one of the easiest and quickest recipes I can think of. The first is something you eat quite mindlessly, the second something you savor with a glass of wine over conversation around the dinner table. The first provides a quick burst of satisfaction with a predictable down soon after, while the second offers a complex, multi-layered, lengthy, and enjoyable experience.

My first escargot-eating experience was when my family had just moved to France. I was eight years old, and my sister was four. It was a cold blustery fall week-end, and we had walked the gardens of the Sun King's castle, the Château de Versailles, on the outskirts of Paris. My sister and I dreaded such walks, finding them exceedingly boring. But the reward was lunch at *La Cuisine Bourgeoise*, a crowded little restaurant right around the corner from the castle, with just a few tables and steamed-up windows. That humble little family restaurant had the best escargots, full of hot green garlicky butter that dripped down our lips and fingers as we dipped small pieces of baguette into the pan after we had pulled the snails from their shells with the help of special tongs and slim two-tined forks and eaten them. I must admit, and my children would agree, that the garlic butter is almost better than the snails, and we would always save the butter dipping ritual for last. My sister would simply order twelve escargots with nothing else before or after, and on the drive home our car would reek of garlic. Such memories remain priceless spiritual nourishment.

The *Slow Food Movement*, whose mission is a cross between "gastronomy and ecology," was founded in Italy in 1986 by Carlo Petrini and has become a worldwide grassroots movement. It inspires us to slow down (the snail is the movement's logo) in reaction to hastily and thoughtlessly ingested *fast food* and put the quality back into what we consume. I have watched the foodie movement take shape at incredible speed in America from the time

I arrived here in 1982 to now. I remember finding skate for a song at a supermarket in Cambridge, where I was living at the time, because nobody knew what it was, and having a hard time finding proper crusty bread during my early years here. Wine was not commonly consumed then. Meanwhile, the number of farmers markets has increased by 370 percent in the past twenty years, from 1,755 nationwide in 1994 to 8,284 in 2014, while retail sales of organic foods increased from $3.6 billion in 1997 to $43.3 billion in 2015, an 1,100-percent increase! Organic farming is one of the fastest growing segments of U.S. agriculture. Between 2005 and 2011, certified organic cropland increased by almost eighty percent. These are impressive statistics attesting to the incredibly rapid and exponential rise in food quality awareness. Not only can I find any kind of ethnic food within an hour's drive of my home, or from my food co-operative, or through the internet, I can find beautiful crusty bread, pasture-raised meat, farm-fresh eggs, local honey, raw milk, beautiful cheeses, and organic vegetables, all from local sources, within twenty minutes of where we live. I am aware that so-called food deserts exist in some urban areas, areas where no fresh food can be found, but as food awareness grows, the availability of fresh foods will keep growing with the demand for it.

As to the celebratory aspect of food, growing up in France and Belgium I got accustomed to three- and four-hour-long meals, Sunday lunches, restaurant outings, business dinners my parents gave at home, and of course holiday celebrations that revolved around special foods. Food is a form of entertainment and enjoyment for me. Today, when we sit with friends or family around a long table with good food and good conversation, I truly live totally in the moment. After the celebration is over, I inevitably realize that I had not thought once of anything other than preparing, sharing, and savoring the meal. This kind of eating nourishes body *and* spirit alike and is the best kind of entertainment to me.

Food reconnects us with our cultural and ethnic food heritage, which is of special significance here in America, where everyone comes from somewhere else. While homogenization of our foods is not a particularly good thing, globalization contributes to the broader availability of specialty and ethnic foods. Nature and humankind are inherently diverse and complex, and so should our foods be. It is beneficial to remember traditional food combinations like the Native American *Three Sisters* corn, beans, and squash, or the corn-bean-lime combination of the South American Indians that assured wholesome and nutritionally complete diets for millennia. Such combinations provide the right balance of amino acids, the body-building blocks of proteins, without having to ingest large quantities of animal protein. That is food wisdom. So is the notion that your own ethnic food heritage, with its specific foods, food combinations, and traditions, may be more in tune with your constitution than the global Western Diet.

The Meat Quandary, The Traditional Diet, and whether it is okay to eat meat without feeling guilty that we are contributing to the demise of the planet

Considering meat eating from an environmental, ethical, and health-related perspective is important in weighing its inclusion in your personal diet. Backtracking our food evolution to the traditional and Paleolithic diets can help to put the meat question into perspective, because both diets have been heralded as potential solutions to our ills. The Paleolithic diet is the one our ancestors consumed prior to the advent of agriculture. This diet resembles what large primates still eat foraged fruits, berries, nuts, greens, roots, mushrooms, and a minimal amount of animal protein. To dispel the myth that the Paleolithic diet consisted of large amounts of roasted meats hunted by he-men, scholar Riane Eisler reports that recent archaeological findings have revealed that "meat eating formed only a minuscule part of the diet of ancestral primates, hominids, and early humans," because "woman the gatherer," rather than "man the hunter," apparently played a much larger role in food acquisition than had previously been recognized. Once our ancestors settled into permanent dwellings and communities about twelve millennia or so ago, and they began to selectively breed annual grain and vegetable varieties, and raise animals as a steady source of protein, our digestive systems gradually adapted to this new so-called "traditional" diet. This is the agricultural diet of annual plants and small amounts of animal meat our digestive systems are currently accustomed to. From its grains evolved the breads, cereals, and pastas we rely on so heavily nowadays.

Attempting to find *the* Traditional Miracle Diet is futile. Author Steve Gagné points out that "neither hunter-gatherers nor agriculturalists can be pigeonholed into a specific dietary category. Diets vary among both modern and ancient groups, with a wide range of foods depending on environment and lifestyle." Take, for example, the extreme diets of the Inuit of the far North, or the Masaai of Eastern Africa. Both thrive on a regimen consisting entirely of protein, marine animal protein and fat in the case of the Inuit, and milk, meat, and blood in the case of the cattle-raising

Masaai, neither of whom suffer from high cholesterol or deficiencies. In fact, their digestive systems might be quite upset by a vegetarian dinner. The Masaai and Inuit diets demonstrate that the human omnivore's digestive systems have always been highly adaptable to whatever grew and flew, or ran or swam locally, even though it may have taken hundreds or even thousands of years of adaptation. On the other end of the spectrum are the Hindus and Jains of India, who have eaten a vegetarian diet for millennia.

Renowned dentist Weston A. Price, who looked into the relationship between tooth decay and the Western diet in the 1930s, concluded that people across the globe who adhered to traditional diets of fresh foods from animals and plants grown in nutrient-rich soils, regardless of which particular traditional diet, not only had healthy teeth but were also healthy in general and had none of what we now call the "maladies of civilization"—heart disease, cancer, and diabetes. This is one more reason, especially in America, to consider your own original ethnic heritage when developing the most beneficial diet for yourself.

Although periods of increased meat consumption have historically been linked to periods of increased brain growth, meat consumption has risen out of proportion over the past two hundred years, though our wisdom has apparently not followed the same trajectory. In conjunction with the population explosion and industrialization of meat *production* (in this term lies the problem) and processing, the exponential rise has had disastrous environmental effects.

Consider that up to thirty-five percent of the world's greenhouse gas emissions are attributed to the meat industry, ahead of those caused by all transportation modes combined, with beef being the biggest culprit, before pork and chicken. More troubling still is that our craving for cheap animal protein at the expense of all reasonable respect for the animals has spun completely out of control in the hands of the meat industry. To safeguard its profit-driven survival, it has shielded itself from public view entirely. Nevertheless, Jonathan Safran Foer has gotten a clear-enough picture of what really goes on behind the scenes, and his book *Eating Animals* is explicit to the point of making me want to cry in exasperation over how low we have sunk to fulfill our combined meat and dollar addiction.

The most glaring issue is that the animals are treated cruelly with a callousness that is hard to believe. They are regularly fed antibiotics (one repercussion of their widespread use and the leaching into our own drinking water is the increasing resilience of certain bacteria and ineffectiveness of some common antibiotics against a number of infections) as a preventive measure to counter the ill effects of, for example, the unnatural grain-based diet fed to cows, which sickens their digestive systems and weakens their overall constitution. Turkeys, chickens, and pigs are overbred for certain characteristics, literally making them unfit for life. The slaughtering process is no less calloused and harrowing. Consult Foer's book for the gruesome, grisly, and absolutely true details. It is chilling to think of the health consequences of eating the meat of these sorry creatures.

On the other hand, what a dramatically different experience might an animal register in its own and our nervous system if it was wild (venison, moose, fish), or pasture raised on its natural diet and slaughtered individually on the farm or a small slaughterhouse by people who respect the animal and are grateful that the animal is giving up its life for our nourishment (as Native Americans might have done). But let's not kid ourselves—if you want to eat meat, animals have to be killed, and try doing that after you have looked into its eyes.

Moreover, our planet is simply not large enough to contain the amount of farmland and water required to raise meat sustainably at the rate the world's population is currently consuming meat. Growing plant-based foods is so much more economical and sustainable, the only viable way to nourish our seven billion inhabitants (and more to come before the population levels off) is to reduce meat consumption drastically if not phase it out altogether. While domesticated animals have been specifically kept as a food source for millennia, besides contributing to a balanced farm environment, the population density in past times was vastly smaller than it is now. You might also ask yourself whether you would eat meat if you had to hunt, kill, and butcher the animal yourself. I think I would become a vegetarian, while my mother has declared that she would rather hunt than forego meat entirely. My husband has been hunting since he was a teenager. Over the past several years, he has gone out regularly in the fall but not brought anything home. I have been wondering whether a shift has occurred in him, a subconscious reluctance to shoot a living being. If you believe it's *just* dead meat, think again.

Eating meat may not necessarily be our main problem, although considering the evolution of consciousness, as I will in Part Three, adds a last layer of complexity to the question. The main problem lies instead in the addiction to ever- increasing *quantities* of meat we have been consuming (to the detriment of our and the environment's health), in the way animals are being

raised in large industrial concentrated animal feeding opera-
tions(CAFOs), in absurd breeding and inhumane living conditions, in the feeding of unnatural diets and medications, in the
environmentally hazardous practices of such facilities, and in the
horrendous slaughtering and processing procedures. Eating
small quantities of wild and pasture or naturally raised meat
from animals treated in respectful and environmentally sustainable ways and slaughtered on the farm or in small slaughter-
houses, or eating sustainably fished wild seafood or seafood from
the few sustainable fish farms, is, and ought to, remain—at least
at this point in our human evolution—a matter of personal taste
and choice. Whether it is morally acceptable to kill an animal for
human consumption to include its protein in your diet remains
your decision under the aforementioned considerations. That
we all have to drastically reduce our meat consumption in general
is a matter of survival for our planet.

The future is never about going backward. Evolution is about
change, adaptation, and added depth and complexity in moving
forward. Our digestive systems have already adapted from the
hunter-gatherer or Paleolithic diet to the traditional one. The
oft-cited and fairly new wheat intolerances that are used sometimes as arguments for returning to the Paleo diet can arguably
be traced to an intolerance to the newer gluten-rich wheat
strains, in combination with the sheer quantities of wheat we
consume in the form of the processed breakfast cereals, pizza,
pasta, pancakes and waffles, bread, and crackers in place of
greens and other vegetables. Going back to the Paleolithic diet
may not be the final answer but a good transition. Waiting for
our bodies' possible adaptation to the Western diet will kill us

before it happens. Any variation on the traditional diet is good if not superior. If, however, we consider our evolution as ongoing and forward moving, it is likely that we will eventually move beyond the traditional diet.

Do we all have to become vegetarians to save the world or avoid cancer?

Tofurky for Thanksgiving? The reactionary flip-side of the meat quandary is a recent trend towards abstaining from meat altogether, fueled by the specter of civilization diseases and the vast damage industrial meat production, and the farmed seafood industry, have wrought on the environment. These are indeed worrisome developments that must be taken into account. Yet we can't demand that all people stop eating meat, period. We have already established that humanity is diverse, that all of us exist at different spiritual levels, and that so much depends on local and ethnic circumstances, customs, and availabilities. Everyone has to decide individually whether or not to eat meat and how the various aspects of the meat quandary apply to them, although the sustainability and addiction factors are essential ones to consider.

Foregoing meat may not be a foolproof prescription against cancer or environmental damage, anyway; the real issue is how much and what kind of meat you consume, if you *do* eat it. Consider that overacidification of the body chemistry through too much refined sugar and carbohydrates (pizza, pasta, bread, baked goods) is a definite factor in tumor formation and all inflammatory conditions. Moreover, as long as crops keep being treated with synthetic fertilizers and chemical pesticides, and as long as we keep ignoring the environmental damage genetically modified produce causes, the benefits of vegetarianism or veganism may not be as clear-cut as we think.

The importance of greens and superfoods

Soil depletion began in the mid-eighteenth century, as mentioned earlier. This depletion of minerals has already had a measurable effect on the foods we eat and, in turn, on our state of mind and well-being. Our food has simply become less nutritious; it has fewer vitamins, minerals, and trace elements than it did in former times. In addition, we are exposed to an increasing array of environmental toxins, which all accumulate in our bodies over time. Thus, returning to grandmother's foods—which has been one of the loudest messages of recent years—may no longer be sufficient to maintain superior health. I believe that our dietary requirements are going through a major shift. We need to relearn to use food as medicine in addition to its primary role as nourishment, we need to supplement, and we need to detoxify. That's where greens and superfoods come in. Greens are our most direct source of converted sun energy in the form of chlorophyll. Large quantities of greens, in the forms of juices or smoothies, or eaten raw or lightly sautéed (not stewed to oblivion), do more than simply alkalize body chemistry. Chlorophyll in large amounts also helps to repair and regenerate body cells, detoxify, and aids in the healing process. Recent research has revealed that the main components of the Western diet—grains, sugar, starch, meat, and fried or heavily cooked foods—acidify body chemistry. This aggravates or causes many of the civilization diseases: cancer, diabetes, some auto-immune conditions, and all inflammatory conditions. Dialing back all these components in your diet, or eliminating them altogether depending on your constitution, can do wonders to alleviate, reverse, or even heal such afflictions.

Superfoods guru David Wolfe has researched foods and supplements that compensate for the shortcomings in our regular food supply. Superfoods are foods that are exceptionally high in antioxidants (environmental toxins can produce free radicals, which antioxidants counter). On Wolfe's list are cacao beans and chocolate (not all chocolate is made equal—the darker the better, because it contains less sugar), goji and golden berries, aloe vera, avocados, hemp seeds and oil, coconut in its many forms, açai and camu camu berries, noni fruit, yacon root, and there are more. Super supplements include AFA blue-green algae and spirulina, marine phytoplankton, kelp, and chlorella, as well as maca powder. Once you have switched over to organics, consider adding some of these into your meals and snacks. Besides better-quality foods, detoxification in the process of cleaning out environmental toxins accumulated over the years, and of reversing calcification. Consult David Wolfe's *Longevity Now* for more information.

Briefly, about peripheral food-related issues

Not only is what you put into your body (or what you *don't* put into your body) important, what you cook and store your food in is, too. Microwaves are out (use your stove and oven), as is anti-stick cookware (seasoned cast iron, stainless steel, and glass are better); plastic food storage containers and plastic water bottles are out (glass, china, and stainless are in); and canned food is out (fresh is best—of all the frozen foods, it seems only berries actually retain most of their nutritional value).

One last consideration. It has been argued that vegetarianism promotes nonviolence. While my brief research into the academic literature on that subject has not conclusively shown a link between vegetarianism and a greater disposition to pacifism, Rudolf Steiner, although no proponent of a vegetarian diet, linked "earthiness" and aggression with increased meat consumption, and spiritual pursuits with a need for a vegetarian diet—which is also the historic reason behind Hindu and Jain vegetarianism. Steiner maintained that, with evolving consciousness, humankind will naturally evolve towards a meat-free diet, a conclusion that sounds plausible to me in light of what I will present in Part Three.

So which diet is best?

My first conclusion is: There is no one-size-fits all diet. Diet is a totally individual thing, based on a combined consideration of ethnic food heritage, constitution, convictions and priorities, age, local food availabilities, health considerations, budget, personal moral convictions, and an individual's developmental, spiritual, and consciousness level.

My second conclusion is that what you eat, and how you eat it, matter. Food is not just *food*. Its quality matters a tremendous lot. Buying fresh and unsprayed food, avoiding feedlot meat, sidestepping processed foods, and cooking from scratch are neither too expensive nor too time-consuming when you consider the question from an insurance perspective. Food can be health insurance for your body and for the environment. The how-to part is about sitting down to regular shared meals, and actually appreciating and savoring the food. My daughter often comments on how good the house smells when I cook, and my husband so enjoys coming home after a busy day to a nicely set table and a tasty, home-cooked meal. This is the part that feeds the soul.

My third conclusion is that it doesn't matter where you begin a deeper inquiry into food. Beginning with baby steps anywhere is fine and is likely to result in further changes down the road.

Finally, I conclude that your improved relationship with food might just change your relationship with your body, the soil and Nature, and perhaps animals.

How to connect more deeply with your food

Observe your body for a few hours after a meal, and become sensitive to how you feel in order to tune into the relationship between the quality of what you put into your body and the quality of what you get out—how much energy and well-being you gain from your foods and beverages. We have a new Tex-Mex take-out place in town, and I've noticed that I feel good, and my stomach feels light, after consuming their food because the ingredients are clean, fresh, and straightforward, and the food is made from scratch. On the other hand, I usually feel discomfort in my stomach and digestive system for hours after eating a fast-food meal or a restaurant meal made with processed foods (this happened to me not long ago after having some nachos covered with a cheesy orange-colored spread). By listening to your body, you will attune to what foods make you feel strong and energetic. Note that the longer the meal sustains you, the more nourishing the food is (high amount of nutritional value relative to the amount of food eaten); the better and lighter your stomach and digestive system feel, the more appropriate the food is for your constitution; and the more energetic you feel after your meal, the closer to Nature the foods are likely to have been.

Instead of following the next fad diet to lose weight, consider eliminating sugar- and flour-based foods for a few months and see what happens. I guarantee that the pounds will melt away as you substitute high-carb for low-carb foods (more greens!), and that your sense of taste will improve. It worked like magic for me.

To continue delving deeper into your relationship with food, select any one topic in this chapter that has perked your interest, positively or negatively, and let yourself be guided from there. Check out the websites in the Appendix. Or get a book from your local library from this chapter's book list, also in the Appendix.

Perhaps you are intrigued to find out more about the problematic meat or fish farming industry. Perhaps the Slow Food movement has a local chapter in your town, or there is a supper club or farm-to-table restaurant in your area like the ones several of our local farms have organized on a monthly basis. Perhaps the idea of eating more locally grown foods is something to start with, which will also lead your awareness to the issue of local economies and the problems connected with globalization. Perhaps you can buy eggs and honey from a neighbor who raises chickens or has bee hives (bee keeping is now approved in New York City, and in Brooklyn some people are beginning to keep backyard chickens, so even when you live in a big city, opportunities exist). Perhaps researching and connecting with your ethnic or cultural food heritage is a meaningful way to begin your deeper connection with food. Food as celebration, the traditional foods of your holidays, is a wonderful topic to get involved in too, perhaps my favorite. Making and sharing meals with friends always leads to good conversation and a sense of belonging and community. I love potlucks because they make gatherings so much easier, but also because of all the interesting recipes that come together. What about growing herbs in window boxes, starting a small vegetable garden, or joining a CSA? The possibilities are endless. Follow your heart and your intuition.

I find meditative joy in preparing food for my family at night. Often I pour myself a glass of wine and lose myself in chopping and cooking, then setting the table nicely. It takes time, yes, but I make choices.

I love food shopping. As a matter of fact, I get more satisfaction out of shopping for food than I do shopping for stuff. Markets are the best. Whenever I travel, I visit markets. They are a feast for the eye, and it is so interesting to see what people from other parts of the world eat.

I express my cultural connections to food in many a meal I cook. Often the French techniques learned during my upbringing bleed through, but I also love Middle Eastern vegetable-and-spice combinations, and Asian tastes. Examine your own ethnic traditions and build on them; make your children aware of them.

The idea is to begin formulating a positive relationship with food. Critiquing what doesn't work, like industrial food or meat production, only goes so far in effecting change in yourself and the culture at large. Voting with your food dollars for what you stand for, and implementing small changes in your personal life, create positive change. Instead of passively watching the Cooking Channel, go into the kitchen and cook. Instead of criticizing the horrific practices of the meat industry, choose to buy less but sustainably raised meat, preferably directly from a farm in your area. Instead of complaining that cooking takes time, reevaluate your priorities and consider cutting time out elsewhere (perhaps some screen time). Live the change you wish to see around you.

Chapter 7

RELATIONSHIPS
AND COMMUNICATION:
WHY TALKING NICE IS SO NICE

"Words can travel thousands of miles.
May my words create mutual understanding and love.
May they be as beautiful as gems,
As lovely as flowers."

—*Thich Nhat Hanh (1926-)*

EEP LIVING ENTAILS A DEEPER AWARENESS OF, and involvement with, everything that pertains to our everyday
life, and so it does with our relationships and how we
communicate with one another. A few years ago, when my then-
fourth grader and I were reviewing her homework, I kept pointing
out the mistakes I found. She first ignored me and then walked
out of the room. On another occasion, my husband observed that
he tends to delete his emails right away and hinted he had lost
some important and much needed information by doing so. I shot

back, "You tend to self-destruct," and dispensed some advice on how he might recuperate the lost information. It went over like a lead balloon.

Children thrive in a classroom environment where the teacher treats them with full respect for who they are despite their age, and who speaks lovingly and compassionately with them. And young learners are very accepting of a teacher's constructive and gently formulated criticism instead of being dressed down for innocent mistakes and made to feel inadequate. Adults are no different. Alan Senauke, a Zen priest, describes the incredibly destructive power of hurtful words and how they resonate on a deep soul level when he says, "Words are like arrows or bullets. Their wounds may be healed, but scars remain." We all know too well how quickly we feel hurt by some thoughtlessly dropped remark about something as minor for example as our appearance ("Well, *that's* a strange looking outfit"). Spoken words can have powerful positive and negative effects, and the way we speak deeply influences our relationships.

What actually went wrong in the two brief exchanges with members of my own family? Deep down they weren't really dialogues but monologues. Both cases might be called instances of *violent communication*. Both are common examples of how we communicate. I viewed the exchange from my perspective, my emotional needs, my beliefs and inner make-up. In the first case, I attacked my daughter by pointing only to the mistakes on her homework and showing no sympathy or offering a solution. I surrendered to an underlying belief that she was not good at math, and I made her feel flustered. Here's a do-over of the dialogue in compassionate terms: "I see some mistakes here. I'm wondering whether you had trouble understanding some of the concepts. Tell me about it. Would it help if we reviewed your homework together?"

In the second case, I judged my husband immediately, professed to know him better than he knew himself, and dispensed unwelcome advice (especially in light of the fact that he is much better at all things technological, and we both know it). Here is a do-over of the second exchange: "What a bummer those emails are gone. Sounds like you lost some information you could have used right now."

Verbal communication goes way beyond the spoken words. In fact, though written words can certainly convey feelings to some extent, and though a telephone conversation provides more clues than an email or a letter, we benefit most from face-to-face communication because we pick up gestures, expressions, emotions, intonation, and body language, which we use as additional clues to interpret the message. Emoticons have become such a rage because texting and emailing prevent us from deciphering the emotional part of the message, and emoticons are an attempt at putting it back in. Understanding fully how the way we speak influences our relationships in both positive and negative ways requires several steps.

Naturally, none of us enjoys being verbally assaulted or emotionally hurt. Yet that's what we do to each other all the time. If I think back and put myself in my daughter's shoes, I get that I attacked and condemned her, that she felt afraid to say she didn't understand the material. And since she is very sensitive, she left the room to avoid being hurt further, and we didn't get any closer to a solution that would have served us both. In the instance with my husband, I offended him too and set up a communication barrier. Both became lose–lose situations.

This sort of communication is a one-way street that builds distrust and misunderstanding because it is not transparent about our underlying emotions and motives. It's not about blame; we simply haven't learned a different way. Most of the time we don't realize what we are doing. We would be at a loss to even put the underlying emotions into words—because we haven't been trained accordingly. It's not part of our culture. Relationships thrive on trust and understanding, or wither in the presence of mistrust and misunderstanding. In our usual ways of talking, we sow much of the latter and not enough of the former.

But there is a better way, and it can put things into a clearer perspective. Several traditions concern themselves with how we speak. Buddhism and Judaism, for example, both have long traditions of teachings on language. In Judaism, hurtful speech is called *Lashon Hara* and comprises all "hurtful speech, which includes gossiping, lying, labeling, judging, scoffing, false manipulative flattery, tattling, and in general speaking negatively of others," Rabbi Joseph Telushkin writes. His practical training proposition is to begin observing your speech one day at a time. He suggests, for starters, choosing one day a month as a "Speak No Evil Day," which can then be expanded to a two-hour period each day, then always on Shabbat dinner.

According to the Buddhist teaching's eight-fold path, *Right Mindfulness* and *Right Thinking,* as the supporting pillars of *Right Speech,* render conversations deeper, more meaningful and more spiritual, in tune with the *other* person. Both lead to *Deep Listening,* a new element that the eminent Buddhist monk, teacher, and writer Thich Nhat Hanh added more recently to the traditional components of Right Speech. Nhat Hanh explains that, if we don't listen deeply and mindfully, we won't talk right and thus won't practice *Right Speech,* because we will speak our own thoughts instead of responding to what the other person is thinking, needing, or feeling. This is what happened in the exchanges with my daughter and my husband. "Deep listening nourishes both speaker and listener," Nhat Hanh points out. My two exchanges clearly did not.

Perhaps the foremost modern-day empathetic communication guru in the West was the late psychologist Marshall Rosenberg, who developed the patterns and methodology of what he calls non-violent communication (NVC), based on his deep understanding of the human psyche. His ideas are not without precedent, having been built directly on the principles of Mahatma Gandhi's non-violence movement and the teachings of its heir, Martin Luther King, Jr. Both of their ideas are clearly recognizable in NVC. Rosenberg translated the principles behind the non-violence movement into the realm of speech by distilling the best of Gandhi and King into NVC's thoroughly comprehensive and convincing methodology. NVC is specific in its approach, and since it is backed by psychological understanding, it features not only explicit techniques but also the deep reasons behind them. This is what makes Rosenberg's method so successful, convincing, and applicable to any situation and under all circumstances—at home or work, in legal mediation and political discourse.

Gandhi recognized that outer refraining from violence ultimately can only come from inner peace and spiritual connection (consider, in this context, the current state of our world). Thus, for Gandhi, inner spiritual maturity expressed itself outward in empathetic action and speech. King furthered Gandhi's legacy of nonviolence by formulating a language of love and compassion. In very general terms, NVC, Right Speech, and *Lashon Hara* all teach that speaking compassionately or from the heart is trainable, and that, simultaneously with making an effort at improving one's speech, at least an inner character strengthening, if not a spiritual maturing, occurs over time. Ghandi and King understood deeply that violence begets violence, and that only internal and external harmony and peace can break the chain of further violence. As King said, "To meet hate with retaliatory hate would do nothing but intensify the existence of evil in the universe. Hate begets hate; violence begets violence; toughness begets greater toughness." Such is the case in restrictive and totalitarian regimes, but also occurs in milder form in many top-down hierarchical and traditional organizations.

Gandhi knew that compassionate speech inevitably leads to deeper human relationships as well as a deeper connection to self. He also recognized that "faking it 'til you make it" is a good way to train the mind to change your own patterns until you can embrace them internally and make them your own. Lastly, he understood that openness, transparency, and truthfulness are crucial elements of nonviolence that build mutual trust in the authenticity of the communication, and that flexibility in communication is vital. "The objective is not to assert propositions, but to create possibilities," he stated. As the lawyer Gandhi was, his ways were those of today's legal mediator, striving towards reconciliation and compromise, which is NVC's goal.

Martin Luther King's message was that love creates spiritual connectedness, hate spiritual disconnectedness, and that they both manifest in the way we speak. Like Gandhi, King had to deal with the general misconception that compassion and non-violence are an expression of cowardice. King taught, "The end of violence or the aftermath is bitterness, [while] the aftermath of non-violence is reconciliation and the creation of beloved community." In complete agreement with Gandhi, he understood the relationship between increasing empathy and an inner spiritual maturing, and the relinquishment, not only of "external physical violence but also [of] internal violence of spirit."

Gandhi and King worked from the outside in, Rosenberg from the inside out. Both ways ultimately go hand in hand and ultimately result in deeper spiritual connection to self and others. You can start on either end; the result is the same. The reciprocity between deeper spiritual connection to self, or Gandhi's increasing absence of inner violence, and an increasingly compassionate way of speaking will become more evident as we move along.

Another example. Upon awakening one morning, my son, still in bed and half asleep, stretched out to his full teenage length with his feet sticking out from under the cover, said to me, "I feel like my blanket is getting too short."

I struck back, "But it's an adult-size blanket, and I am not buying a new one."

Say what? Had he just asked me to buy him a new blanket? No. I was reading into it, all the while listening to my own narrative. Instead of addressing his need for warm feet and offering empathy for his cold feet, I reacted from my perspective of family budgeter-in-chief and justified why he wasn't going to get a new blanket—a response clearly devoid of connection. If I had reacted with compassion and a smidgen of understanding of where my son was coming from, I might have replied, "I see that your feet are sticking out. They must be getting cold. How about I tuck them back in?"

Marshall Rosenberg's premise is that our widespread cultural separatedness from spirit, and thus self, is also reflected in our current way of communicating with one another. As a matter of fact, Rosenberg goes so far as to say, "The language of our culture prevents us from knowing our Divine Energy more intimately, that our language makes spiritual connection hard."

Susan Gillis Chapman, a more recent author on compassionate communication, puts it less spiritually and more culturally: "Our communication patterns contribute to creating our social environment. An angry person lives in an angry world and a generous person lives in a generous world."

Rosenberg's background in psychology helped him to develop his method of nonviolent communication. I share his belief that "spirituality is at the base of nonviolent communication," and that a more conscious empathetic choice of communication inevitably leads to deeper spiritual connection to self and others. Thus, the deeper our spiritual connection or maturity, the more gentle and compassionate our verbal communication patterns become. We need to get away from the *me* perspective, from *what's-in-it-for-me*, which creates a lot of pain, hurt, misunderstanding, and aggression. Chapman argues, "Me-first thinking is supported by a culture of mistrust, the message that it's not safe to be vulnerable." We judge others way too easily. Judgments come from assumptions based on deeply held beliefs and are me-based. My own deep-rooted belief held that my daughter was not good at math. It was clearly a me-based judgment, because she has since become an "A" math student. Compassionate communication, on the other hand, is *we* based, which creates win–win situations all around.

On a different note, could it be that our culturally negative-oriented thinking, as I explored in detail in Part One, conjures up exactly all the negative stuff we fear, that we dwell on and that we speak about, but are trying so hard to actually avoid? What would happen if we expressed positive thoughts, spoke out about how we *do* want things, how we *do* want to be treated? What a difference between "Don't talk to me like that" and "I feel hurt when you use such harsh words." Expressing what we actually feel is one of the many things Rosenberg's method teaches. He flips our perspective from negative-oriented to positive-oriented in his communication model, which is what I am trying to do in this entire book—to shift your perspective to what you *do* want and away from what you *don't*.

In addition to empathizing with the other person first, Rosenberg therefore directs our minds towards the positive, to expressing how we'd like to be treated and spoken to (not how we *don't* want to be treated and spoken to). The idea is to give, in order to get, by trying to understand how *the other person* feels and what *she* needs; to lend a compassionate ear and empathize, and to get a friendly, mutually acceptable response in return. Moreover, his method trains us to listen deeply into ourselves by acknowledging and recognizing our own feelings and emotions. In our present communication patterns, our emotional needs remain hidden: They are implied but not spoken. So, in a seemingly contradictory way, perhaps surprisingly so, the effect of our present language is the exact opposite of what we are trying to achieve. When feelings and needs remain hidden and unacknowledged, they emerge in unexpected and unpleasant ways, as hurt feelings and misunderstandings. The result of practicing NVC is more depth—in understanding the other person, because we attempt to define what feelings and needs originated her reaction; in understanding ourselves, because we attempt to understand our own needs and feelings and what originated them. NVC is thus based on straightforwardness and honesty with ourselves and our communication partner. It is deep communication, spiritual communication, empathetic communication —it is communicating *with* the other person, not *against, besides, over,* or *without* the other person. Ghandi scholar V. V. Ramana Murti summarizes it like this: "The way of violence works as a monologue, but the nature of non-violence is a dialogue." Rosenberg's goal was to create dialogue and peace instead of fighting violence. Therein lies the fundamental difference.

Two further important principles relate to compassionate communication. The first is that we all have common needs, physical and emotional ones. In addition to needs relative to physical sustenance (such as food, health, and air), we have needs relative to security (such as peace, safety, and protection), connection (such as love, harmony, and companionship), and meaning (such as creativity, purpose, and growth). Take some time to digest the full list of Universal Human Needs, Emotions, and Feelings, which was put together by BayNVC and is reprinted here in Appendix B, to understand how deeply true they ring, and how little they are acknowledged in our culture. Wouldn't it be wonderful if we all recognized that kindness, nurturing, purpose, or inspiration are universal human needs, and helped each other to attain them? And what about power, space, or trusting? So many,

many people on this Earth enjoy none of that. And many others could have more of their needs met but are simply unaware of them, have not been taught—neither was I until I took a NVC seminar.

The second fundamental principle is that we can use our emotions as gauges or indicators to measure whether, and to what extent, those universal needs that have particular personal meaning to us have or have not been met. Esther and Jerry Hicks present a list of emotions in scale form, from best to worst, in their book *Ask And It Is Given*. On the top of the scale are high-frequency emotions such as joy, passion, and enthusiasm; the emotions travel down in frequency through boredom and disappointment, and end with the negative and low-frequency ones like worry, anger, revenge, and hatred, with fear, depression, despair, and powerlessness at the very bottom. The higher on the scale the emotions are that you are feeling, the better your needs are being met and the more connected you are to your spiritual self; the lower on the scale, the less those needs are being met, and the more disconnected from your spiritual self you are.

We are ill trained in our culture to express what we are feeling, even to choose the right word for each thing we are feeling, and to make use of this information. If we were better at it, our relationships would be better, and there would be fewer misunderstandings, grudges, and hurt feelings. In order to use compassionate communication effectively, we need to train ourselves, first to acknowledge, and then to name all these emotions. Heidi Feichtinger writes, "Emotions are the language of the heart, words are the language of the head." When we drop from the head into the heart, we become compassionate. Let these descriptive words for emotions sink into your mind: *giddy, tickled, rejuvenated,* and *elated,* but also *mistrustful, displeased, regretful,* and *nostalgic,* and finally *heavy-hearted, wretched, agitated, helpless, terrified, repulsed,* and *fragile.* Merely becoming aware of them and being able to put the different feeling gradations into words opens up communication possibilities. Wouldn't you love to feel giddy with excitement? Or jubilant at news you've just received? I feel troubled by a lot of what I read in the news, and sleepy when my head sinks into the pillow at night. I also feel horrified about the realities of the industrial meat industry and alarmed at the inaction of our politicians in dealing with climate change. See the range of feeling words I've just presented?

In spiritual terms, all this translates into the following: the better we know how to meet our needs and the more of our needs are being met, the more positive our emotions are and the more spiritually connected we become to self and spirit. This literally makes us more fulfilled. Compassionate communication is a vehicle for recognizing, acknowledging, and working with these two elements—needs and emotions—and expressing them in our language. It follows that our internal degree of presence or absence of spirituality manifests in the way we speak. Nurturing successful friendships and relationships, personal and in business, has everything to do with how deeply we are in touch with ourselves. Writes Arielle Ford, author of *Wabi Sabi Love,* "Before you can tune in to your partner's reality, you first have to learn how to tune in to yourself."

Here's one more example. Several years ago, my daughter dawdled over finishing her milk at breakfast when we needed to meet the school bus. I was briefly patient but ended up shouting.

What would a more compassionate exchange have looked like? "I see that your glass is still full, and I'm nervous because the school bus is going to get here in five minutes. I need you to finish your milk right now so you can catch the bus." Although more wordy, it becomes a more truthful way of speaking that lacks insinuated requests and inferred feelings. Along the way we learn to exhibit flexibility, in that we do not demand action from our partner but ask for a consideration of our own position, with the understanding that the other person has freedom of choice and might consider acting out of empathy and compassion for us.

The last major communication process to deepening relationships is *listening* with empathy and compassion, which is about setting aside our own narrative and actually tuning into our partner's message. Such attentiveness is the thrust of Thich Nhat Hanh's *Deep Listening* I mentioned earlier, and Marshall Rosenberg's *empathic listening*. Putting ourselves in our partner's shoes makes for truly mindful listening. So often we brush over what someone says, only to insert our own experience, the *me*-perspective:

> *You:* "I broke my toe yesterday."
>
> *Me:* "Oh, no—that happened to *me* last year. And
> you know what, my doctor...blah, blah, blah."

Instead, consider:

> *You:* "I broke my toe yesterday."
>
> *Me:* "Oh, no, you must be in pain. What hap-
> pened? Tell me about it."

By studying compassionate communication, I have realized how thoroughly, perhaps how perfectly, our inner workings, our consciousness, are interwoven with our language. It is not new to me to recognize my deeper self and others' deeper selves in our outward physical manifestations, such as those I explored in Part One. What I eat reflects my inner thinking, my convictions. That I refrain from eating processed foods, and cook from scratch with pesticide-free ingredients, directly reflects my beliefs. My beliefs express themselves on the physical plane through my behavior. I recognize in other peoples' activities what they are about on the inside, in their consciousness. Everything we believe reflects on the material plane—in what we wear, how we manage our finances, what work we do, how we manage our bodies, and so on.

Not only do we reveal our innermost workings like an open book in everything we do and how we do it, we also reveal them in our language. We cannot hide our innermost workings. They are there for the world to hear, although not everyone is able to interpret the message. Our degree of spirituality emerges in the way we speak and communicate. The more compassionate our language becomes, the deeper our connection to self and spirit is, and the deeper and more harmonious our relationships with others become.

Although Adele Faber and Elaine Mazlish published the groundbreaking *How To Talk So Kids Will Listen & Listen So Kids Will Talk* in 1980, not until Rosenberg did anyone develop a structured, psychologically based method of analyzing, understanding, and cultivating our speech patterns with the direct intent of improving our relationships.

To set the record straight, NVC, or *compassionate communication* (the affirmative is always preferable to the negative), is not about getting someone to do what you want her to do! That is what our present way of communicating is about. NVC is about *connection.* This is why NVC is quite wordy, since it involves teasing out where your partner comes from emotionally, where you come from emotionally, and how to meet in the middle. Someone in my NVC workshop spoke of a partner who had retorted to an attempt at communicating compassionately, "Don't NVC me." Ultimately, NVC is about creating win–win situations through potential compromise, because that is what it takes for a successful relationship.

To illustrate the full extent of how differently NVC works, let me describe a major conflict I mediated between my children a few years ago. It took quite a while, twenty-five minutes or so, in part because it leaves the involved parties a lot of reflection time should they need it. It was summertime, we had meant to go to the beach the previous day, the outing had not worked out, and I'd promised the children we could go the following day. But the following day turned out to be really chilly and breezy. My son, who is almost four years older than his sister, switched gears easily and proposed we check out the new supermarket instead. My daughter, on the other hand, was devastated and accused me of breaking a promise, which I had—under attenuating circumstances. My son tried to persuade his sister, but she wouldn't hear the weather argument. She simply felt crushed and cried. So I backed up and gathered all my newly won skills. First, I restated both positions and the fact that the weather was lousy for a beach outing, but offered the coupon for free ice cream at the new supermarket as an incentive to alter her stance. I got no reaction from her. I turned to empathy. I asked whether she felt devastated, disappointed, and that she couldn't trust me. This lasted for at least ten minutes. She needed a lot of compassion. Yet she still could not bring herself to shift. I restated that the two of us would just have to go to the cold and windy beach alone if there was no movement from her side; her brother did not want to come. On the other hand, we could always go to the beach another day, while having ice cream and a look at the new supermarket today. That would be a win–win situation for her, since she would get both, beach and ice cream, albeit on two different days.

After more time to think, a shift occurred, and it was agreed that we would do ice cream today and the beach on the next warm day. I felt very successful and satisfied that I had been able to apply so many different NVC skills—empathic listening, empathy giving, time to reflect, and asking as opposed to demanding a shift. As John Gray wrote in *Men Are From Mars, Women Are From Venus*, "If I seek to fulfill my own needs at the expense of my partner, we are sure to experience unhappiness, resentment, and conflict. The secret of forming successful relationships is for both partners to win."

Our present culture is spiritually disconnected. The unseen has been ignored and reasoned away because of our single-minded focus on the physical, that which we can know with our five senses. As such, our needs, emotions, and beliefs run as an *undercurrent* in our language. They remain inferred, not spoken, and the disconnect shows up in our language in general in the form of judgments, insinuated demands, negative feelings, impatience, and unmet needs, like a chronic disease. NVC as a deep or spiritual language unearths these elements and puts them right on the table. It is a sincere and truthful way of speaking that acknowledges the feelings and needs in all of us. Through its techniques, compassionate communication makes it possible to create win–

win situations for both parties. Along the way, we gain depth in relationships by understanding the other person's feelings, and we give back by revealing our own feelings, as opposed to letting people guess what they might be. We listen deeply and connect in a much better way. In the end we learn self-compassion and genuine connection to self, spirit, and others. This is spiritual communication. Thich Nhat Hanh, says it like this: "Speech is the way for our thinking to express itself aloud. Our thoughts are no longer our private possessions. We give earphones to others and allow them to hear the audiotape that is playing in our mind." He emphasizes that our innermost thoughts, our subconscious, our values and beliefs, our education and culture, all become apparent in our speech. Our choice of words, our way of addressing people, our ways to express ourselves in general, are all noticeable in our speech, and our communication partners register this information on a soul level. It seems that the harsher and more aggressively we communicate, the more spiritually disconnected we are from self and others; the more gentle, harmonious, and compassionate our way of speaking is, the more connected we are to our own inner spirituality and that of others. We could also simply say that we are more or less in tune with ourself and others. The quality of our speech reflects our level of inner spiritual maturity, which in turn influences the degree of compassion and connection we are able to offer our partners. Words can hurt, and words can heal.

One last thought: the male, or *yang* element, outweighs the female, or *yin,* in our present culture, a point I will pick up in Part Three. In that regard John Gray writes, "Martians [i.e., meaning men] have a win-lose philosophy—I want to win, and I don't care if you lose." In NVC, we try to fix this imbalance. According to

Marshall Rosenberg, speaking is "more than a communication process. . .it's really an attempt to manifest our spirituality." Nhat Hanh clarifies this idea: "Words can create happiness and suffering," and "they can give someone a complex, take away their purpose in life, or even drive them to suicide." Applying the precepts of compassionate communication, on the other hand, we are able to promote and create happiness, harmony, win–win situations, and a deep and loving connection to our partners.

Where to start to begin communicating more compassionately

A heads-up: This has been, and remains, the most difficult area of change for me personally because of the surrounding culture. You won't find many good examples to follow and are pretty much on your own until you can find a few like-minded people. The mantra is awareness, then practice, practice, and more practice.

Keep a journal for a week or two, and record short passages of dialogues from your daily work or home life to reflect on. This is where my examples come from. When you read back what you said and how a dialogue unfolded, you have time to reflect on how to make it better next time.

Take an NVC workshop in your area to learn the techniques from the professionals.

Join a local practice group that meets regularly.

Practice listening deeply—watch your partner, look into her face, tune out your own narrative, and forget about thinking what your next reply might be. Put yourself into your partner's shoes.

How might she feel right now? What does she need?

Stop yourself from responding according to the *me-too pattern* when your partner talks about an experience. Instead, respond directly to what your partner actually said.

Before making a request ("I need that report by 4:00 p.m. on Thursday") think of the outcome you are looking for, then put it into a suggestion, not a demand, such as: "We have that big presentation on Friday, remember? Could you rearrange your schedule so that your report might be ready by 4:00 p.m. on Thursday? That would really help me out." (Yes, NVC is more wordy). How could anyone not respond "Of course" to that nice request?

When your partner hurls a hurtful remark at you ("Where did you get *that* haircut?") or demands action ("I told you I needed that data *now!*"), pause and try to define what emotions come up for you—then put them into words. In reply to the haircut remark: "Sounds like you don't like my new haircut. I feel hurt when you say that, because I actually quite like it." And in reply to the demand: "I feel pressured by your demanding tone, but your boss is probably breathing down your neck. Let me get you that answer right away."

Chapter 8

THE BODY, AND A NEW WAY
TO HEAL

*"Current medical explanations for health and disease are cultur-
ally driven, and. . .we cannot separate biology from culture."*

—*Lewis Mehl-Madrona, MD*
(1954–)

*"If what we have been calling 'mind' and 'body' are really one, then
all diseases, without exception, are and must be 'psychosomatic'."*

—*David Michael Kleinberg-Levin*
(1939–)

I DID NOT FEEL I MATTERED in her assembly-line practice. Then I began to wonder aloud why childbirth was relegated to the hospital; it's not an illness, after all. The doctor cited "risk," especially in "older" women, implying deterioration of the body with age as a given. I was thirty-seven when I gave birth to my first child and did not feel "older." The constant doctor visits in a clinical environment, and the various tests, made me paranoid. Instead of ensuring I was well, they kept looking for symptoms. A few years later, during labor with my second child, I had a stuffy nose due to a cold, which made those breathing techniques I was being asked to perform, impossible. The nurses refused to give me decongestant nose drops, mumbling about possible interferences and side effects, although they would have given me an epidural with potentially really serious side effects without hesitation. Doubts about the whole medical model began to set in.

Deep Living is about digging deeper, and so it goes with understanding the body and how we heal.

Health and the healing process, and shift to a new model

In Part One we explored the idea that healing is much more than "fighting illness," that it is a process of inner transformation, and that it doesn't follow a predictable cookie-cutter course because everyone is unique. Physician and author Marcey Shapiro stresses that illness is not a punishment but a "communication of a misunderstanding." In German you ask someone who is not well, *"Was fehlt Dir?"* or "What are you lacking?" Since healing means "to become whole," we are missing an aspect of ourselves when we are not whole, when we are out of balance or ill. When we are healed, or whole, we are complete—nothing is missing or lacking. However, simply by virtue of being incarnate in a body and living a dualistic existence, we will always be working on overcoming polarity.

Healing is a complex process that the mainstream medical community does not quite understand because scientists have not truly studied it. The current Western medical paradigm is pathology oriented and reactive, thereby focusing on what's wrong and treating symptoms rather than studying what being well means and how the healing process functions. We take notice when there is a symptom, then look for ways to get rid of it—aspirin for a headache, cortisone or steroids for an inflammatory condition, antibiotics for a bacterial affliction. Pharmaceuticals can indeed be very effective and life saving. Allopathic or Western medicine has its strengths, such as in emergency and trauma medicine, in treating infectious and acute conditions, providing joint replacements, and performing cosmetic and reconstructive surgery. On the other hand, it does not as successfully treat mental illness, chronic and auto-immune diseases, viral infections, allergies, or cancer.

For the past three hundred years, scientists have believed that, if science can only go deep and far enough into the furthest reaches of the universe, or into ever-more microscopic sub-atomic or sub-cellular depths, we would eventually find final answers to everything—and prove along the way that there is a rational scientific explanation to all life processes. Under the mechanistic interpretation of the body that arose from this scientific approach, we believe that the body breaks down over time and deteriorates, the way machines do. We transferred thinking related to mechanics and machines to the human body, and machines cannot heal themselves.

But the ongoing compartmentalization of the human body into separate parts—i.e., eyes, heart, lungs—and the increasing specialization of the medical disciplines—i.e., ophtalmologist, cardiologist, pulmonologist—have prevented us from keeping the forest in sight. Instead, we have spent three centuries analyzing the trees, their leaves, their cells, and their sub-atomic parts. This prevents us from acquiring a holistic understanding of the interrelationships of all body components—and seeing the mind's role in it.

Especially with advancing age, we take illness instead of radiant health for granted, because we believe that deterioration and decline are the inevitable stage that precedes death.

But could that view simply be an artifact of the underlying belief system? Sure, historically, life expectancy has increased considerably. But let's face it—old age is often overshadowed by chronic and debilitating conditions that are kept at bay with the help of pharmaceuticals, though never truly healed.

Yet we know so much more now about nutrition as well as the body's physical and mental needs to remain in excellent health. I'm not claiming that our bodies will become immortal if we change our belief system, but we can surely do better than taking it for granted that we will become pill- and doctor- dependent as we grow older, or believing that auto-immune and chronic conditions are incurable.

Baseline well-being

Some fundamentals bear repeating to create a baseline for understanding the complexity of health. Good food (not just good tasting but actually healthy, restorative, and nourishing), sunshine (aka vitamin D), movement, adequate rest, and as few toxins as possible assure a good foundation for a healthy body and create the basis for emotional well-being—or is it the other way around? Which came first, emotional or physical well-being? Positive thoughts and beliefs, and meeting our need for love, respect, dignity, safety, trust, and creative expression ground us and create a healthy emotional foundation for taking aspirations beyond the basics of mere survival and toward the qualities that make us human. Both kinds of well-being, the physical and emotional, are prerequisites for good health. But while both inform and influence each other, the more basic physical ones, according to Maslow's hierarchy of needs, must be met before we can ascend and aspire to higher emotional and spiritual goals. If I am struggling to make ends meet and put food on my table, I am not in a frame of mind to meditate or inspect my potentially negative belief system. Once we meet these foundational needs, we can further develop the emotional and spiritual side, which in turn sets the stage for even better physical health.

A different model, the one underlying Asian healing modalities, is proactive and wellness-oriented. It is energy- based and works on the premise that an organism is constantly adjusting and self-healing, and that energy blockages cause imbalances and afflictions. We have all seen pictures of elderly Chinese practicing qi-gong or tai-chi in public squares as preventive health measures and know that you can practice yoga until the day you die. Pioneering holistic physician Andrew Weil writes in his book *Spontaneous Healing* that the difference between East and West is healing from within versus treating from the outside. His simple-sounding prescription for good health is in line with the idea that we need to evolve—from the premise of treating symptoms when it is already too late, to one that focuses on leading a preventive lifestyle that involves healthy eating, getting rest and movement, cultivating a healthy mind, and avoiding toxins.

Historical and cultural context of health and healing

To put things into perspective let's take a look at our ideas on health and healing since we adopted Newtonian thinking. These ideas are greatly shaped by the prevailing culture. When cultural beliefs change, so does our understanding of how to heal, including the methods we use to facilitate the healing process. Conversely, when we as a culture collectively change our understanding of human existence, health, and healing, medicine and its procedures change as well. David Michael Kleinberg-Levin, Professor Emeritus of Philosophy at Northwestern University, wrote in a seminal 1990 paper, "The history of medicine is inseparable from the fact that there have been, and still are, many different, often conflicting representations of the human body."

Rembrandt's famous 1632 painting *The Anatomy Lesson of Dr. Nicolaes Tulp* illustrates how the medical exploration of the human body began with dissection and took us gradually from the outside in, from a strictly mechanical study, through a biochemical understanding of the body's processes, to acknowledging that the mind somehow also seems involved in our well-being or absence thereof. However, we have not yet dared to bring this thought process to its logical conclusion. In the Western world we are still healing the body separately from the mind. In a nutshell, psychology and psychiatry have been treating the mind, allopathy the body. The fact that we have separate disciplines for body and mind is due to the belief, now fraying at the edges, that the world is a purely physical manifestation. We have understood body and mind as separate, and the mind as an aspect of the body with seat in the brain. While we are in the process of shifting towards a more integrative understanding, the mainstream is still quite ensconced in what Larry Dossey, another philosopher doctor, calls brain–body medicine, because we as a culture don't seem quite ready to consider that the mind might inform the body and not vice versa. But, as Kleinberg-

Levin makes clear, "It is impossible to delineate the end of psychology and the beginning of biology. Does it not follow that the boundary between body and environment is also indistinct?"

The mechanistic type of medicine we have practiced for the past few hundred years manipulates the physical body and has evolved from blood letting and leeching to surgery, MRIs, and an array of other invasive procedures. In *Reinventing Medicine,* Dossey points to a crucial shift in our belief system that this era has caused. Prior to this time, he writes, "People did not expect medicine to deliver cures." The insight that the body can he healed is huge and reassuring. With the shift to the biochemical body model, we included vaccines and drugs in our toolbox, which influence the body's biochemistry and have achieved some amazing results, albeit usually with unwanted side effects, besides masking symptoms without truly healing the underlying condition, as is often the case, for example, with chemotherapy. Moreover, this shift also rapidly resulted in the widespread and erroneous conclusion that modern medicine is so powerful it can vanquish *all* afflictions with its methods. It encouraged our adulation of the doctors as gods in white coats.

When this turned out not to be true, when we began to seek second opinions because we found that there was room for interpretation of symptoms and proposed therapies, when we realized that numerous conditions did not respond predictably to standard treatments, we entered the era of brain–body medicine. According to Dossey, this began after World War II as an extension of what was then called "psychosomatic illness," which means an affliction fabricated by the mind. During this current and ongoing transition phase of brain-body medicine, mind and body modalities are often combined in treating the patient, as, for example, in the pairing of conventional cancer treatment with meditation.

The medical community has been circling the involvement of the mind in illness, health, healing, and wellness for over a century and has given the various approaches that acknowledge that our mind somehow plays a role in becoming ill fancy names like "psychoneuroimmunology," "behavioral medicine," "psychology and psychiatry," "mind-body medicine," "psychosomatic illness," "conscious intentionality," and "biofeedback." Dossey says our resistance to trusting the mind lies in having to acknowledge and process what we can't see, and trying not to call what's happening in the mind *consciousness*, because we are still attached to the brain. As we move into a new medical era and a holistically inclusive and consciousness-based healing model, we find the need to "look under the hood," as author Cheryl Richardson puts it. That means that we need to inspect how the mind functions and how thoughts and beliefs influence the body and the world at large. We realize that, for example, ADHD/ADD or depression originate in the mind, but the mainstream is still treating them both with suppressive pharmaceuticals because we have not yet found a better way.

Once we can let go of our attachment to the brain, we will enter what Dossey calls the "era of non-local medicine." Cell biologist Bruce Lipton thinks that the shift in belief from genetically predetermined, victimized biochemical humans to co-creative, empowered individuals will be as enormous as the shift in belief from a flat to a round Earth. When we finally recognize ourselves as spiritual beings in a physical body, we will devise modalities that heal the mind so the body can heal itself. This will be a monumental consciousness shift, away from high-tech, high-cost medicine to low-tech and low-cost methods, which we are already seeing in many alternative modalities such as kinesiology, homeopathy, reiki, healing with food, and the like. These methods can be powerful, and the cost only involves the practitioner's time.

Larry Dossey is suggesting that the incoming era of non-local medicine will provide us with another cure, the one for our present all-pervasive cultural fear of death, because a non-local mind exists beyond the physical body. Then we will understand French philosopher Pierre Teilhard de Chardin's famous observation that "we are not human beings having a spiritual experience, but spiritual beings having a human experience." Kleinberg-Levin takes the dissolution of the mind–body dualism to an integrated whole between body, consciousness, environment, and culture to the next level, a human being who is an integral part of the whole grand creation.

When we and our environment and our surrounding culture and fellow men become one, when we recognize that we are all part of the same field of consciousness, we will finally come to grasp that we are in this together. A relevant example: Many of the Western civilization diseases have sprung from an unhealthy and unnatural lifestyle we have adopted together as a culture, like, poignantly, the Western diet—high in sugar, meat, refined carbohydrates, chemicals, and grains, and low in greens and other vegetables, vitamins, and minerals—which makes so many people sick. We need to heal this destructive behavior together and collectively.

The significance of the underlying cultural story is important, and the story you personally subscribe to is crucial to the effectiveness of any given healing modality. Lewis Mehl-Madrona, the Native American doctor, psychiatrist, and author whose healing approach is cultural context-oriented, argues in *Narrative Medicine* that, if the patient is not convinced by the doctor's "healing story," she won't follow the treatment. As he says, "Healing rises or falls on the quality of the story, not the modalities chosen."

This means that what's important isn't the healing modality you choose, but that you believe the healing modality you choose is the best one to help you heal, and that you trust the practitioner. After my pregnancies, I no longer bought the Western story about health and illness. I lost trust because I found too many contradictions, too many inconsistencies, too many unanswered questions in it. How do you explain spontaneous remission? How do you rationalize the placebo and nocebo effects? How do you justify accidents? Why do two people with the same diagnosis and therapy heal differently, or that one of them lives while the other dies? Why do some children inoculated with the DPT vaccine still get pertussis? Why was it that, while two-thirds of the European population succumbed to the bubonic plague, one-third survived? What made the survivors different?

The power of your thoughts and self-healing

We are quick to go to the doctor when a symptom arises, and ask for help. However, we concluded in Part One that doctors, procedures, and pills are only props that set into motion, and support, the body's own inherent healing abilities—although healing itself involves an internal mental process or activation set into motion through our own intent and will power, which assist the healing mechanism. Dossey writes in *Meaning and Medicine* that all psychic healing is spontaneous self-healing in reality, although the presence of an external "healer" can "potentiate" the self-healing effect or speed. My own homeopathic physician, Michele Galante, says that "doctors provide an illusion of help." So the intent, the will to heal, must come from within; then the healing process is potentiated through props, procedures, and doctors, as well as psychological support from community, doctor, and family.

Much has been written about the power of positive thinking and its flipside, the effects stress and negative emotions have on the body. But medical research has not yet dared to reverse the question and ask whether, and how, intentionality and belief changes can actually heal. That is because the potential sponsors of such research don't believe they do and would find it risky and irresponsible to create studies that assigned one half of a test cohort with a certain affliction to allopathic treatment, and the other cohort to healing with intent, positive beliefs, and emotional support. The contradiction in this is that we entirely trust ourselves and our bodies to heal colds or broken bones, and do so without a second thought. Why, then, do we believe the process can be effective only in those cases but not in others, like cancer or autoimmune disorders? If we can make ourselves ill, we should be able to reverse the process unless the body has deteriorated to the point of no return.

Mainstream science has neither studied, nor developed proper methodologies for such a belief-change therapy, even though alternative practitioners have, and there is already a body of literature on the subject.

Then there is the question of responsibility. People have a

problem assuming responsibility. It's easier to blame something or someone else. It's easier to look for the cause outside yourself and place the healing responsibility in someone else's hands, those of the "experts." As a culture we would find it irrational under the present belief system to assume responsibility for self-healing cancer or diabetes. We don't even assign the responsibility for healing the cold or broken leg to ourselves, even if we firmly believe that both can be healed easily. But is there a universal healing law, or isn't there? After all, we believe in the Law of Gravity every time and always, not just sometimes.

In *Train Your Mind Change Your Brain,* science writer Sharon Begley reported on neuroscientific research that has shown shifting beliefs actually change our brain structure, which demonstrates that our thinking manifests in physical form. That is also what cell biologist Bruce Lipton's research has shown. He writes, in *The Biology of Belief,* "The fact is that harnessing the power of your mind can be *more* effective than the drugs you have been programmed to believe you need. The research I discussed. . .found that energy is a *more* efficient means of affecting matter than chemicals." However, the power of positive thinking only cures if subconscious countervailing and sabotaging beliefs are reprogrammed. It's a tenet of current conventional thinking, for example, that genes determine our biology and predispose us to certain conditions. But, Lipton asserts, "It is not our genes but our beliefs that control our lives." He speculates that the placebo effect has deliberately been swept under the table, not only because of dogmatic Newtonian thinking, but for financial reasons. Thinking yourself well is low-tech and unprofitable. Lipton stresses the power of placebos and cites as an example the proven ineffectiveness of antidepressant drugs and, for that matter, the relative effectiveness of placebo pills to treat depression. Going further into our microbiology, he asserts that our personality or self, our consciousness, resides in each cell of our body, and that "the brain controls the behavior of the body's cells." It has been well publicized that organ-transplant patients often undergo personality changes, which an acquaintance of mine, whose husband had a heart transplant several years ago, has confirmed.

The flipside of positive thinking, negative and self-sabotaging thinking, causes the reverse of the placebo effect, the so-called "nocebo effect," which demonstrates the power of negative thinking. Negative thinking adversely affects your health, and can do so to such an extent as to become fatal. If, for instance, you are diagnosed with stage-4 cancer, firmly believe that it is untreatable, and your doctor tells you so as well (and you believe your doctor), it becomes a fatal diagnosis or self-fulfilling prophecy: You believe yourself to death. Doctors, as well as our surrounding culture, possess incredible powers of negative suggestion, which can deeply undermine our ability to heal. The crux of the problem, according to Deepak Chopra, is actually to "know" the diagnosis of an illness. For that reason, a homeopathic practitioner refrains from naming afflictions, concentrating instead on mental and physical symptoms. Our bodies are able to cure broken bones because we "know" that the body can cure them. Cancer has not been treated convincingly within the Western medical model. So being given a diagnosis of that disease sets the mind up for failure. In his introduction to *Quantum Healing*, Chopra argues that several of his practice's terminal cancer patients have recovered completely, and he sees it as proof that "the mind can go deep enough to change the very patterns that design the body." Anita Moorjani, now an author and inspirational speaker, is another one who recovered completely from end-stage Hodgkin lymphoma after her organs had already shut down. You can listen to her tell her story at anitamoorjani.com.

What is the difference between our ability to heal a broken bone or cancer? Our belief system.

Another scientist who has done very convincing research into the power of our beliefs regarding the physiology of the body is Ellen Langer, a Harvard social psychologist. She conducted a now famous study on nursing home residents in 1979, who, for a short time, lived in a setting that modeled the 1950s. The startling finding of the study was that the physical and psychological effects of aging were reversed in a measurable way due to immersion in the earlier time period, when the subjects had been twenty-five years younger. The results were published in book form for the general public in *Counter Clockwise*. While Langer's study focused more specifically on the *physical* effects of aging and the potential to reverse them, it also demonstrated convincingly how thinking and consciousness affect the physical body in the most direct way. She currently has a study underway on stage-4 breast cancer patients, which I believe will become a landmark study. Two other persuasive studies document actual cures as a consequence of intentional mental techniques. One describes the cure of irritable bowel syndrome through guided imagery; the other describes successful placebo surgery in patients with arthritic knees.

The late research scientist Valerie Hunt wrote, in her *Infinite Mind*, "Inner healing focuses on belief systems as the contaminating source." With regard to the powerful influence of the beliefs of our surrounding culture, Hunt says, "Belief systems that are firmly ingrained culturally take on the power of absolute law." Deepak Chopra maintains that there really are no limitations of the mind, will, and consciousness to cure disease. According to him, state of mind is crucial, since anxious states of mind, *actual belief in the sickness*, "sends out the neuro-peptides associated with negative emotions, these latch onto the immune cells, and the immune response loses its efficiency."

Quantum Physics/Quantum Healing

While we distinguish thought from matter in our dualistic universe, in a quantum reality there is a fluid boundary between them because they are made of the same stuff, which is energy. In an energetic universe, physical and spiritual, mind and matter, thoughts, beliefs, values, and culture, all exist as one undivided whole. We need to recognize our embeddedness in culture and environment, and understand that the body is an energy system that is part of a bigger energy system. Things we eat, think, feel—our body itself—all have a particular energetic frequency, as do the people and things we surround ourselves with. Everything influences everything else reciprocally; as Chief Seattle purportedly put it, "Whatever you do the web, you do to yourself." Someone who is depressed and despondent has a very low frequency, someone exuberant and radiant is very high on the frequency scale, and they can both take you either up or down with them.

Acknowledging and shifting away from negative thoughts—generally seeing every glass as half empty, or believing that everyone is out to get you—is one of the most important ways to clean up your mind, and that will improve your life and your health tremendously, as it will the lives of those who interact with you. Valerie Hunt has said that we are each responsible for healing ourselves because our ill health influences those we interact with so tremendously that one could say that it's irresponsible to be sick. If you are unhealthy or ill, if you are unhappy or find yourself surrounded by negative people, if you don't love what you do, acknowledge it and *do* something about it. You are not a victim. Negative thoughts and beliefs reduce your energy frequency—we are healthy above 62 mHz—and with it your ability to heal. You attract the energy that you put out. If you send out negative vibes, you get back low-frequency vibes and will therefore believe that the world is negative when it is actually you who are. On the other hand, when you are excited and passionate, happy to be alive, you will attract more of the same higher frequencies. That is what "like attracts like" is about.

Moreover, your beliefs and thoughts shape your tomorrow. If you think negative thoughts today, your future will be negative. Guaranteed. You can change that today by making an effort to see the world through rosier glasses. And if you keep thinking the same thoughts today that you did yesterday, your future will look like today. If you don't like what you see today, you need to shift your thinking today for a different tomorrow.

The good thing, actually the utterly fabulous thing, is that you can fake it 'til you make it. Inspect your beliefs about health and healing. Do you actually believe that any condition can be healed? Do you believe that you can and are worthy of radiant health? And what are you doing today to create that radiant health for tomorrow? Is you glass still half full? Are you surrounded by a vibrant circle of friends? Do you have access to wonderfully healthful foods? Are your basic material needs taken care of, and then some?

Chopra defines quantum healing as "the ability of one mode of consciousness (the mind) to spontaneously correct the mistakes in another mode of consciousness (the body)," although there are some limitations such as depletion of inner abilities (as in chronic diseases or old age). While quantum physics does not *per se* prove consciousness, the electro-magnetic or quantum physical explanation of where and how healing can happen touches on the interconnectedness of everything. It is a timely theory as we begin to shift from seeing the human species as a mere physical phenomenon to seeing it as entangled in an electro-magnetic energetic world that integrates spirit and matter. In one sentence, cell biologist Bruce Lipton summarizes this view as follows: "The universe is *one indivisible, dynamic whole* in which energy and matter are so deeply entangled it is impossible to consider them as independent elements." In fact, Lipton concludes, "energy and matter are one and the same."

Thus, thoughts and beliefs possess the same energetic quality that energy-healing modalities like homeopathy, acupuncture, reiki, and others manipulate within the body's electro-magnetic system. In that regard, thoughts and beliefs, as well as the various energy healing modalities, all influence the life-force body's energy stream. Lipton explains that disease first manifests at this molecular energetic level and only later in the physical. He says, "The behavior of energy waves is important for biomedicine because vibrational frequencies can alter the physical and chemical properties of an atom as surely as physical signals like histamine and estrogen." This echoes Hunt's observation that "healing occurs through changes in the electromagnetic field." And, Marcey Shapiro points out, "All illness begins in the realm of energy disruptions. . . . All healing begins in the realm of energy rebalancing." Lipton calls for a biology that integrates both quantum and Newtonian mechanics, because the manifestation of a disease begins at the molecular or quantum level before it becomes apparent at the macro or Newtonian medical level. When Bernie Siegel, the alternative heart doctor of the 1980s, said that unconditional love is the most powerful stimulant for the immune system, he was already promoting our embeddedness in a quantum universe.

We are groping for patterns and reasons, such as heredity and genetics, environmental toxins, and diet. But we firmly believe in "accidents," like breaking a leg or being involved in a car crash, as a chance encounter that happens for no particular reason. And we "fight battles with cancer," refuse to take responsibility for our bodies and minds, and don't, at least in general, acknowledge our embeddedness in, and reciprocal relationship with, the unseen aspect of our existence, that world which quantum physics says interacts with, and is the same as, the material world.

Many healing modalities operate on this quantum level. The only one that does not is the Western allopathic model. All others—Ayurveda, acupuncture, reiki, qi-gong, voodoo, prayer, distance healing, and many more—are systems that manipulate the electromagnetic energy of our bodies in various ways, in the direction of rebalancing or towards imbalance, as the martial arts or voodoo, for example, can do.

I concluded in previous chapters that one-size-fits-all solutions are inadequate because we are neither machines nor statistics; they are equally inadequate for agricultural systems, for diets, and for healing mechanisms and modalities, because we are all unique and circumstances are all unique. Since each person's personal context and history, health circumstances, and cultural milieu are entirely unique, the healing mode ought to be entirely custom tailored to each individual. That leaves you to figure out how to mobilize your particular inherent healing capacities. Perhaps in the future there will be consultants in the medical community who are qualified to match you with the best practitioner and healing modality for your circumstances and beliefs. For now, there aren't.

We need to combine Eastern and Western healing approaches, energetic and allopathic healing modalities, Newtonian and quantum approaches, to achieve more comprehensive effects. As Hunt puts it, "Outer healing [allopathic] saves the biological life, while inner healing [energetic or electro-magnetic] focuses on belief systems as the contaminating source." In acknowledging that allopathic techniques have limitations, we open the possibilities for alternative and complementary healing modalities and can use them to best effect.

Like a math equation that always needs to remain balanced between the left and right side of the equal sign lest it become incorrect because it is out of balance, we need to keep a balance within ourselves—body and mind together. The German expression *"Was fehlt Dir?"* that I alluded to earlier in this book is an expression of the need to reestablish harmony where something is amiss, where the energy has been disrupted, where an imbalance has occurred. The simplest example might be noticing that you are tired, the body's message that you need rest. Once you have slept you have reestablished balance in your body—which illustrates how a symptom or illness is not a punishment but the body's way to communicate a deficiency. When you develop a fever in response to a viral infection, the fever's purpose is, similarly, to make the bodily environment inhospitable and kill the virus. When we look at symptoms or illness from that perspective, it becomes clear that they are indications of underlying processes that are sending a signal and attempting to reestablish balance. It's your body talking to you, demanding attention. If you are in touch with your mind and body on an ongoing basis and respond to small signals, you can reestablish balance before the symptoms become more pronounced. If you ignore these little symptoms, the bell will begin to ring louder.

How do you personally heal?

I was always looking for quick answers and thought that the next author or healer would have a magic solution to solve all my problems pronto—whether it was Gary Craig's *Emotional Freedom Technique*, Alexander Loyd's *The Healing Codes*, Henry Grayson's *Use Your Body to Heal Your Mind*, or Esther and Jerry Hicks' *Ask And It Is Given*. But magic without personal involvement doesn't happen. It's a process. With a mental shift, however, almost anything can happen, and quickly, as it does in spontaneous remissions.

Which cultural health and healing story do you personally subscribe to? What does health mean to you? How do you heal? How much responsibility are you willing to take for your well-being? Personal involvement in the healing process is vital to true healing. As Bruce Lipton writes, "Using prescription drugs to silence a body's symptoms enables us to ignore personal involve-ment we may have with the onset of those symptoms. The over-use of prescription drugs provides a vacation from personal responsibility."

Because health and healing are very complex matters, because the answers are not simple, because you are not a statistic but a unique individual, and because you are embedded in a particular cultural belief system, persistent self-inquiry and a willingness to open up and change are important in custom- tailoring a healing plan for yourself. A body snaps at its weakest link. What is yours? A professional reading of your astrological profile by a reputable astrologist can help if you have absolutely no idea.

Here are some thoughts about digging deeper in the areas that make up your health profile. Books and books have been written about each of the aforementioned topics, so this is only a sum-mary of where and how to start.

1. Eat good food

What do you eat and drink? The most important thing about creating fabulous health is to become aware of what you put into your body, how you react to foods and drinks, and to consider an external (what foods and drinks you buy) and internal (removing toxins, adding supplements) clean-up if necessary. Food and drink are what nourish you and build new cells. Garbage in, garbage out—GIGO, the acronym that originated as an explana-tion of how computers malfunction—also applies to your body. If you feed your body sugar, pizza, soft drinks, and processed foods, how can your body give you back radiant health? You can't make leather shoes out of plastic, or a silk dress out of nylon, or create radiant health from inferior food. Superior nourishment is the very best health insurance you can buy. All books by David Wolfe are a good start if you are interested in digging deeper into nutrition, as are the titles listed in the suggested reading list for Chapter 6.

While diet is a very individual thing—our digestive systems are not made alike—in very broad strokes we can all benefit from eating more greens and less sugar, more vegetables and fewer high-carb foods, drinking more water and tea and less alcohol (wine, especially red, is good in reasonable amounts, hard liquor not so much), soft drinks and juices, and eating less meat and more plant-based foods. The quality of your food makes a huge difference in your energy level, disposition, and bodily ability to self-heal. Why not keep a journal about how your body feels after eating certain foods or certain meals? How do you react to them? How do you assess your energy? How does your stomach area feel after a meal? How is your digestion? Does your breakfast take you all the way to lunch without having to resort to a soft drink or a donut as a pick-me-up in mid-morning? Do you have cravings? Sugar crashes? You should see a direct relationship between food intake and energy level.

Decrease your sugar intake; change to natural sweeteners. Slowly switch over to buying organic, non-GMO, non-irradiated food. If you eat meat and eggs, do so from small local farms; buy wild caught fish and raw dairy products. Decrease meat, and increase plant-based foods. Consider adding more vegetables to your diet, as well as fish oil and chlorella supplements because even organic soils are depleted these days.

2. Cultivate positive thoughts

Next in the line-up of basics is the cultivation of positive thoughts and wholesome beliefs. They're as important for good health as proper nourishment, and they're free. If your beliefs and thoughts run rampant, remain unexamined, and turn out to be self-sabotaging, they could damage your well-being. Bruce Lipton's *The Biology of Belief*; *Ask And It Is Given,* by Ester and Jerry Hicks; and *Use Your Body To Heal Your Mind,* by Henry Grayson, are good starters into the subject. Ask yourself about your relationships. Do you have many friends? Do you eat meals in company? Do you have a significant other? It has been well documented that people with a solid social network live longer, and that people who eat in company are happier. Other questions to ask yourself and write journal entries about include whether you love what you do for a living. If not, you may need to "look under the hood." Do you experience stress in your life? What does it stem from? Do you love your life? What parts of it do you not like? What do those parts you don't like show you? Inspect your underlying beliefs and how you talk to yourself.

3. Give yourself rest and exercise

Time out in fresh air and Nature, as well as physical exercise, should be no-brainers, but, chasing the next buck in our busy lives, we tend to forget about them. Often these elements are last on the list. For exercise a walk in Nature is more beneficial than running on a treadmill under fluorescent lights in a gym. Chopping wood, mowing your lawn, and yoga are all great for mind and body.

The gist of successful movement is to engage in it often and outside, rather than inside and in strenuous sporadic spurts. If you can incorporate movement into your daily routine—going dancing, gardening, or walking to work, instead of spending extra time for exercise—it won't feel like a chore on the to-do list. Read Joan Vernikos's *Sitting Kills, Moving Heals* on the basics of the importance of movement, and don't stop your kids from fidgeting. Fidgeting is actually good for you.

Getting adequate amounts of sleep, and leaving the electronics out of the bedroom, are also important. The body heals during sleep, when the cells repair themselves. Too little sleep, and the self-healing gets interrupted.

4. Eliminate toxins

This is a big deal, because toxins lurk everywhere. They abound in the industrialized world we have created for ourselves. Whether in the form of amalgam tooth fillings, radon in your basement, pesticide residue on conventional produce, fire retardant in your couch, pollution in the air you breathe, off-gassing of carpets in your apartment, harsh chemicals in your cleaning products and cosmetics, or chlorine in your drinking, shower, or pool water, they are everywhere and accumulate in your body over the years. Read David Wolfe's *Longevity Now* on how to clean your body of toxins, and Sloan Barnett's *Green Goes With Everything* on how to clean your house.

Take it slowly if you are new to this detective work, and begin in one area—say, your household cleaners. Take any one of them (Windex, toilet bowl cleaner, oven cleaner) and replace it with a do-it-yourself version you can readily find on the internet. Many of them involve nothing more than baking soda and white vinegar and are a lot cheaper than the toxic commercial versions. What you can't easily make at home, you can buy in a non-toxic version.

Move on to your personal care products, such as shampoo and conditioner, lotion, mouthwash, shaving cream, hair dye, cosmetics and what have you. Online databases like ewg.org and safecosmetics.org are very helpful. Every time you're out of something, replace it with a non-toxic product; that way the switch is less daunting.

If you live in a city with chlorinated and fluoridated tap water, install a water filter. If you live in the country and have well water, install a filter to avoid pesticide and chemical residue, radon, and who knows what else. As David Wolfe says, "Buy a filter, or be the filter."

Replace pharmaceuticals to the extent possible with natural remedies and therapies. Look into herbs, homeopathy, essential oils, and superfoods. Have your amalgam fillings removed.

Purchase household goods, such as linens, rugs and carpeting, mattresses, and curtains that are made from natural materials. Inspect sofa-stuffing flame retardants—most of them are toxic.

Avoid buying drinking water that has been stored in plastic bottles, and use reusable glass or stainless steel bottles when you go hiking or to the gym. Store leftover food in glass, not plastic. I save wide-mouthed glass jars and reuse them for food storage. Avoid aluminum cookware; switch to high-grade stainless steel (preferably, Saladmaster), enameled cast iron, glassware, or cast iron.

Buy organic foods to avoid ingesting pesticide residue; alternatively, wash your conventional produce thoroughly in a home-made vegetable wash. Ditch your microwave oven.

In most cases healing is a gradual process. We heal in stages, climbing up a ladder so to speak. David Hawkins, a physician and psychiatrist, as well as Valerie Hunt, relate this ascension to gradually increasing our individual and collective energetic frequency or energetic vibrational levels. A certain level of unawareness, for example, will be apparent and shine through across the board in areas such as the quality of relationships, of how we communicate, of our beliefs and thoughts, of how we interact with our environment—in short, it will show in everything we do, speak, and think. So physical illness is not the only indicator of the individual developmental level. A rise in overall consciousness or energetic frequency level, as David Hawkins explains it, reverberates across the entire human being, not only in the physical or the emotional body. Because of this interconnectedness, we can begin to heal on any level or aspect, and changes on other levels will ensue. It is a complex, multi-layered, and individual process. Start anywhere. Start with any subject that speaks to you, that you connect with naturally. As I mentioned previosuly, a healer once told me I needed to connect more with Nature and recommended I get a tree identification book. I was a bit skeptical but did so, and the book has been sitting on my bookshelf ever since. A tree book was not the best way for me to connect with Nature. Food is my thing, because I grew up in a food culture; so that is where I started. Through food and cooking, I dove into a deeper relationship with Nature and farming, and with myself via nutrition and understanding how we heal with foods that are right for us or how those that aren't can make us ill; it is through food and reading about practices of the commercial meat industry that I understand better how much I love animals and experience how it becomes harder and harder for me to eat meat. Look for any other area that calls out to you, and begin there.

One last thought: Read, read, read about health and healing; talk, talk, talk to many different practitioners. Hear what they have to say, how you feel in their presence. Whom do you trust? Do you feel heard? Has that person had the time to listen to you? Do you resonate with the modality they offer?

PART THREE

The Bigger Picture,
And Why All of This
Is Really Important

*"No problem can be solved from the same
level of consciousness that created it."*

—Albert Einstein (1879–1955)

*"The key to growth is the introduction of
higher dimensions of consciousness into our
awareness."*

—Lao Tzu (sixth century BC)

Chapter 9

A BROADER PERSPECTIVE

Y OU GAIN AN UTTERLY DIFFERENT PERSPECTIVE of New York when you look down on it from the Empire State Building on a clear day, or of the surrounding landscape from the top of a mountain, than when you are down "in the gully," walking the streets between tall buildings, or hiking through the woods.

For me there is comfort in knowing of a bigger picture, and in the case of our cultural and environmental crisis, a bigger picture can provide assurance that what we perceive as chaos at the street level may very well have a reason, purpose, or explanation on a higher level. As my yoga teacher said recently, "Chaos is order without predictability." We may not be able to spot the coherence from our perspective, but it's got to be there somewhere deep down. From down in the streets of our Western culture, it can be difficult to realize that we have options, that the way we live individually can be changed, that a culture is not static and can change. That is why traveling is so eye opening. It leads you to compare. And knowledge of the mechanism of how reality, your life, and your culture get shaped, as I suggested in Part One—gives you the power to redefine things for yourself instead of being swept away in the wave of other people's cultural thoughts and beliefs.

Recently a friend switched jobs because she felt so stressed by her manager's negative and discouraging behavior towards her. Two weeks into her new job, she exclaimed, almost in disbelief, "My new boss just told me I'm brilliant!" The former manager had a negative attitude that tinted everything in her life, including her assessment of my friend's performance. The new manager's joyful disposition led to a diametrically opposed evaluation of the same person's competence. So what you perceive as real depends, not only on your perspective, but on your inner make-up, and that in turn depends on how your brain is wired, which can change slowly over time but also suddenly.

In earlier eras we perceived the world differently than we do now. At one time we believed so firmly that the Earth was at the center of the universe that we burned Giordano Bruno at the stake for saying otherwise. Our consciousness, individual and collective, is not static; it changes and evolves, opening up new vistas on how we perceive our world. Evolution is the gradual and cumulative change of organisms over long periods of time, layering on complexity along the way. Not only does your physical body change over time, your consciousness evolves as well. In fact, it is your evolving consciousness that drives the growth and development of the brain, nervous system, and body. Neuropsychologist and consciousness researcher Allan Coombs explains that hand in hand with "increasing physical complexity of an organism" goes an "enlargement and improvement of the nervous system," which deepens the organism's consciousness at the same time. So with increasing development of consciousness we, individually and as a collective, gain deeper awareness and lucidity. On the other hand, until we reach a certain consciousness level, there are things that simply remain hidden from us, that we are unable to comprehend or see until we reach a higher level of awareness. You may have heard of the story of the Indians, true or not, who were unable to see Columbus's ships appearing on the horizon because ships did not exist in their minds. And children are not interested in the wider perspective of their surrounding world until their rational minds begin to develop. Our minds open up magically with increasing awareness, lucidity, and tuning into the metaphysical as we proceed on our spiritual journeys and reveal things that simply did not exist, or so we believed, previously.

We are now picking up the thread from Part One, where I showed, with the help of the house example, that consciousness shapes matter, which means that our thoughts, beliefs and ideas, propelled by a sufficient amount of creative energy, create physical things and the life around us, and not vice versa. And if our consciousness is not static—as we just saw—but evolves, then we shape, not only our personal lives, but our culture and its development as well. It follows that *our culture is an expression of our individual and collective consciousness level.*

Allan Combs points out that it was Georg Friedrich Hegel, the German philosopher, who first formulated the idea of "human consciousness developing through historical progression and leading to increasingly higher forms of expression." Hegel's theory inspired several later thinkers, among them Henri Bergson, Pierre Teilhard de Chardin, and Jean Gebser in Europe, and Sri Aurobindo in India, into pursuing and refining the idea of a gradual evolution of consciousness. More recently, Ken Wilber developed a complex consciousness evolution theory in this country, and cell biologist Bruce Lipton writes, "The story of evolution is. . .the story of ascension to higher awareness." Eastern philosophies, too, speak of such an evolution towards greater spirituality. In a nutshell, they are saying that we not only progress in our awareness individually over time, but humanity's combined consciousness develops and evolves as well, expressing itself in culture. Swiss philosopher Jean Gebser was called a *cultural anthropologist* for unraveling the consciousness evolution process backwards. By deduction, he unearthed earlier consciousness structures from the evidence of historical events, ideas, and manifestations.

This book is about imbuing life with meaning, putting the present Western existential crisis into perspective, and helping you to rebalance your life in an effort to move our cultural and spiritual evolution forward. It is an effort to inspire the rebalancing of your priorities and aspirations away from a culture that lopsidedly leans towards quantification, materialism, science, and scientism, as well as male dominance (another effect of imbalance I will soon address), and towards a culture that is more quality oriented, more spiritually oriented, and more partnership oriented.

In Part Two I inspected the *small* picture, how we can change our personal relationships with Nature, agriculture, food, speech, and our body to improve the quality of our personal lives, and how these personal interactions reverberate and in turn shape and create the surrounding culture. By becoming aware of our values and beliefs, and actively shaping them instead of simply adopting those of the surrounding culture, "because that's the way things are," we play an active part in rebalancing ourselves and our culture and advancing our spiritual development. As Arne Naess has said, life is about self-realization. Bedogne formulates it differently: that we, and life, naturally strive for perfection. In that regard our culture becomes more balanced or more perfect, the more balanced or more perfect we as individuals become.

As a species we are part of a much bigger picture, embedded in and part of life on planet Earth and the cosmos, continuously changing, adapting, evolving and maturing. Part Three of this book is about the opportunity to see our present cultural malaise and environmental crisis against the backdrop of an evolving consciousness and culture. Many believe that we have begun transitioning to a new structure of consciousness. What we observe as doubts, frustrations, crises, and regressive attempts at taking refuge in former more traditional cultural expressions can also be seen as a questioning and breaking down of the old patterns. We can interpret the widespread freedom movements, the Occupy movement, and the global grassroots movements for a sustainable lifestyle as early episodes in the birth of cultural renewal. Understanding this relationship helps to see the present situation, not as a doomed world gone bad, but as a stage in a larger evolutionary scheme and an opportunity to embrace this shift without resistance, instead participating with passion and co-creating for a better tomorrow.

A new and improved consciousness

The more speculative and esoteric accounts of a historic consciousness evolution mostly derive their insights from introspection, while the more grounded academic versions are based on scientific research and academic extrapolation. However, these descriptions do all point in the same general direction, towards an emerging culture that is more cooperative, more co-creative, and more partnership-oriented. Despite all the graphic violence depicted in the media every day and the extremely violent reality of the early twentieth century, Harvard psychologist Steven Pinker has documented in his recent book *The Better Angels of Our Nature* that we actually live in the most peaceful period of humanity yet. He diligently documents the dramatic decline in violence over the course of human history to prove his point, although as a down-to-earth evolutionary psychologist Pinker points to reason, not an evolving consciousness, as the cause behind this hopeful trend.

If mind shapes matter, and if our increasingly complex human consciousness has actually shaped history over time, then historical events, trends, and tendencies, as well as thought movements, would be an expression of our collective consciousness and its developmental level. As Gebser has surmised, they would be the outer physical expression of how our minds worked in those earlier times. Author and scholar Riane Eisler revealed evidence in her 1987 book *The Chalice and the Blade* that pre-Neolithic cultures were more sacred- and goddess-oriented, and that they were partnership-oriented compared to later cultures. After the Neolithic, Western societies took a dramatic turn towards male-dominant cultural models in which aggression, domination, and violence became typical. Pre-Neolithic cultures employed technology for creative and lifestyle-enhancing purposes, instead of the violence-oriented resort to domination and warfare in the later cultures. Interestingly, all this evidence remained hidden until recently because our male anthropologists interpreted the evidence from within their dominator model paradigm. According to Eisler, there have been slight historic fluctuations in the degree of male dominance. But she detects a more pronounced shift towards greater balance between male and female, beginning in the nineteenth century with greater women's empowerment and the abolishment of slavery, followed by the mid-twentieth century nonviolence and race equality movements, and most recently the fall of the Berlin Wall and the Iron Curtain in 1989, and the Arab Spring and Occupy Wall Street movements in 2011.

To add two more voices to this trend, sociologist Paul Ray and psychologist Sherry Anderson considered, in *The Cultural Creatives,* published in 2000, how this new consciousness expresses itself in the lives and culture of a quarter of the adult American population, about fifty million people, and about eighty million Europeans. Cultural Creatives embrace what the authors call "authenticity," and which I call "holistic" or "spiritual," and their lifestyles reflect all the quality-oriented trends we visited in Part Two. Economist and cultural visionary Jeremy Rifkin has been talking about the trend to a more cooperative and less destructive culture for decades in his many books, notably *The Empathic Civilization, The Third Industrial Revolution,* and *The Zero Marginal Cost Society.* Europeans seem to have been more receptive to his message than Americans, and he has been advising many European leaders on issues ranging from economy to climate change and energy.

Back to Riane Eisler, though, whose theory complements, not only what some of the more esoteric thinkers have written, but also what many contemporary scientists are seeing and saying. While Eisler's report is based strictly on extrapolation from archeological evidence and scholarly interpretation, spiritual thinkers like Sri Aurobindo, Teilhard de Chardin, Gebser, and Steiner have used introspection to gain insight into the history of consciousness. In broad strokes, and without going into the differences among their respective theories, these thinkers maintain that our consciousness has evolved from an earlier, simpler group consciousness and is moving towards an increasingly subtle and complex consciousness as well as greater spirituality. According to them, human consciousness was sleep- or dreamlike in its earliest stages, but about a hundred thousand years ago humanity passed a threshold into self-awareness, a developmental step each of us still experiences around age three when we become aware of the "I." Our time perception was different in earlier times as well. Supposedly, we went from a complete absence of time perception through a circular understanding of time (thinking according to natural cycles, as some indigenous people still do) to the linear time perception we developed around twenty-five hundred years ago in conjunction with the rational analytical thinking pattern that is still in effect today but apparently crumbling.

It was actually Einstein who made us aware of the relativity of our kind of time perception when he spoke about time turning in on itself, stretching and contracting (we experience that on a perceptual level when we feel time flying or something taking forever), and the possibility of observing earlier time periods on Earth if, speculatively, one flew far enough away from our planet and looked at it from over there.

From the consciousness evolution perspective, the development of spoken language (it is disputed when this arose) and written language (about five thousand years ago) were subsequent

externalizations of an inner consciousness awakening and the be-
ginnings of the distinction between inner and outer worlds, and
spirit and matter, as Coombs, Lachman, Chardin, and others have
explained. In the Neolithic period, the concept of polarity, or the
perception of opposites as such, arose around the same time in
which Eisler sees the slow and steady shift from goddess-oriented
partnership cultures towards the male-dominated hierarchical cultures that have prevailed ever since. Not only were societies partnership-oriented before and up to the Neolithic, they also did not
perceive opposites as we now do. People, Eisler explains, lived in
a holistic world with a more dreamlike consciousness state than
present consciousness structures allow. Historians have actually
pointed out that a different consciousness structure, a different
way of thinking, began to shine through ancient Greek philosophy
as compared to writings of earlier times. That was when our present rational thought system developed, which only spread to the
rest of the Western world during the Renaissance.

So both systems, the evidence-oriented academic, and the in-
trospection-oriented philosophic, point to this earlier dreamlike
state. It is possible that the "undivided native mind" we now ad-
mire in indigenous people, their greater partnership with Nature,
is indicative of an earlier pattern of consciousness than our own
in the industrialized North.

To return to the possibility of a newly emerging consciousness,
the New Physics (now a hundred years old), and Chaos Theory,
also point to a new perception of reality, away from the separation
of matter and spirit and towards an understanding of an energetic
whole. Some of the scientists who have recently espoused this new
understanding of reality, and whose names I have already men-

tioned, include Bruce Lipton, Fritjof Capra, pharmacologist Candace Pert, Humberto Maturana, Francisco Varela, Rupert Sheldrake, and Deepak Chopra. Their theories all point towards an integral or holistic reality in which all is energy and no actual distinction exists between matter and spirit—the former simply a solidified form of the latter, both constructed of the same essence.

In our present culture, the male side, the physical, the rational, the yang, is favored and more pronounced, and this lopsidedness between the feminine and the masculine causes the cultural stress we are currently feeling. The new consciousness structure, it is anticipated, will not only balance the two aspects of our reality better (i.e., the physical and the metaphysical), it will go further. It will maintain and build on the rational analytical thinking abilities we have incorporated into our consciousness but also include the spiritual aspect we currently lack. In that respect we will rise above what may perhaps have sounded earlier like a glorification of the undivided native mind. From this broader perspective we can regard our economic, cultural, and environmental crisis in a more positive light. Though we have temporarily left the spiritual by the wayside, this may perhaps be a necessary hiatus in order to better refine our rational capacities.

Conclusion

There is no such thing as a return to a "more innocent past," and Muammar Qaddafi's recent fate illustrates the futility of resisting a trend toward greater momentum rather than accepting it and going with the flow, the driving tenet of Taoism.

If "life is what your thoughts make it," as Roman philosopher emperor Marcus Aurelius is reported to have said, then we must think those thoughts that create the life we want to live—and by this I mean, not only the one we want to experience *personally*, but also what we want our collective future, and that of our children and grandchildren, to look like.

While many indications point to a larger picture of an evolving human consciousness and a newly emergent framework for it that may be more balanced, more partnership-oriented and more spiritual, it is vitally important that we are part and parcel of this development and help shape it. Instead of resisting it (as in efforts to return to a more fundamentalist lifestyle), or passively letting it happen, it is much more rewarding to embrace it and even make it happen through active involvement. At this stage in our consciousness, it is important to take responsibility for our destiny. As soon as we wake up individually and emerge from unawareness, we must own that. When John F. Kennedy said so aptly, "Ask not what your country can do for you, but what you can do for your country," he was pointing to this very destiny.

There can be no blanket recommendation on how you need to live your life. There is no *right* or *wrong* way. Your life reflects your individual awareness and consciousness as much as the consciousness of the culture it is embedded in, since both are entwined. Although a leap of faith into the unknown is always scary, the beautiful thing is that life becomes better and better, more meaningful, and more fulfilling as consciousness evolves. Nature is complex and diverse, and so are you. You are a unique and special case, and so should your life be. Reach, then, into your heart and feel what makes you happy and fulfilled. We take life too seriously, and I am no exception. If we played it more like a game of personal fulfillment than a chore to make the next buck (or the next PTA meeting, or the next gym session), we would be a lot happier.

Many have written about the changes that are already happening, and the more radical changes that still need to be made to prevent a global environmental suicide or economic collapse. Many have pointed out as well that no one knows whether these developments will be peaceful and gradual, or cataclysmic and painful. Once we awaken to the realization that change is inevitable, that we need to own our evolution and that of our social matrix, we must embrace this progress. Progress and evolution are not only inevitable, they are also about moving to a higher level without losing the insights previously gained. The more we all embrace and participate and *are* the change, the more peaceful and gradual it will be.

I believe that the next step in humanity's maturing consciousness is a return to a greater invitation of the spiritual into our lives without the loss of the analytical thinking capacities we have acquired over the past twenty-five hundred years. When we truly listen to our hearts, we won't go to war any longer, yell at our children, put harmful foods into our bodies, spray poison on our soil, or rape Nature. And as Riane Eisler has pointed out, we will use science and technology for life-enhancing purposes, to further our self-realization and fulfillment. Instead of the usual win–lose scenarios, we will create win–win game plans that are environmentally sustainable and socially just, good, not for some, but for all.

Appendix A

Suggested Further Reading By Chapter Subject

Part One

Chapter 1

Fritjof Capra, *The Hidden Connections*

Huston Smith, *Why Religion Matters*

Chapter 2

Charles Eisenstein, *The Ascent of Humanity*

Thorwald Dethlefsen, *Schicksal als Chance*

Chapter 3

Deepak Chopra, *Ageless Body, Timeless Mind*

Roger Eastman, Ed., *The Ways of Religion*

Valerie Hunt, *Infinite Mind*

Bruce Lipton, *The Biology of Belief*

Lewis Mehl-Madrona, *Narrative Medicine*

Candace Pert, *Molecules of Emotion*

Part Two

Chapter 4

Alan Drengson, Ed., *The Deep Ecology Movement*

Charles Eisenstein, *Sacred Economics*

Fons Elders, Ed., *Visions of Nature*

Paul Hawken, *Natural Capitalism*

Rob Hopkins, *The Transition Handbook*

James Lovelock, *The Gaia Principle*

Bill Plotkin, *Nature and the Human Soul*

Jeremy Rifkin, *The Third Industrial Revolution; The Empathic Civilization*

David Suzuki, *Wisdom of the Elders; The Sacred Balance*

Dr. Seuss, *The Lorax*

deepecology.org

earthday.org

environmentalhistory.org

sierraclub.org

transitionculture.org

transitionus.org

Chapter 5

Lisa Hamilton, *Deeply Rooted*

Fred Kirschenmann, *Cultivating an Ecological Consciousness*

Charles Mann, *1491*

Bill Mollison, An *Introduction to Permaculture*

Rudolf Steiner, *Agriculture Course: The Birth of the Biodynamic Method*

Keith Stewart, *It's a Long Road to a Tomato*

biodynamics.com

permaculture.org

Chapter 6

Colin Campbell, *The China Study*

Masaru Emoto, *The Miracle of Water; The Healing*

Power of Water

Sally Fallon, *Nourishing Traditions*

Steve Gagné, *Food Energetics*

Marion Nestlé, *What to Eat*

Michael Pollan, *In Defense of Food; The Omnivore's Dilemma*

Jonathan Safran Foer, *Eating Animals*

Will Tuttle, *The World Peace Diet*

David Wolfe, *Longevity Now; Superfoods*

Otto Wolff, *What Are We Really Eating?*

slowfood.com

slowfoodusa.org

Chapter 7

Susan Gillis Chapman, *The Five Keys to Mindful Communication*

Arielle Ford, *Wabi Sabi Love*

John Gray, *Men Are From Mars, Women Are from Venus*

Thich Nhat Hanh, *The Art of Communicating; Anger: Wisdom for Cooling the Flames*

Esther and Jerry Hicks, *Ask and It Is Given*

Adele Faber and Elaine Mazlish, *How to Talk so Kids Will Listen and Listen So Kids Will Talk*

Marshall Rosenberg, *Nonviolent Communication*

cnvc.org

Chapter 8

Sharon Begley, *Train Your Mind Change Your Brain*

Daniel Benor, *Consciousness, Bioenergy and Healing*

Deepak Chopra, M.D., *Quantum Healing; Ageless Body Timeless Mind*

Thomas Cowan, M.D., *The Fourfold Path to Healing*

Thorwald Dethlefsen, *Krankheit als Weg*

Harry Dienstfrey, *Where the Mind Meets the Body*

Larry Dossey, M.D., *One Mind; Reinventing Medicine; Healing Beyond The Body; Meaning and Medicine*

Henry Grayson, *Use Your Body to Heal Your Mind*

Steven Hodes, M.D., *Meta-Physician on Call For Better Health*

Ellen Langer, *Counter Clockwise*

Marcey Shapiro, M.D., *Transforming the Nature of Health*

Bernie Siegel, M.D. *Love, Medicine and Miracles; Peace, Love, and Healing*

Sloan, Barnett, *Green Goes With Everything*

William Stewart, M.D., *Deep Medicine*

Andrew Weill, M.D., *Spontaneous Healing*

ewg.org

safecosmetics.org

Part Three

Chapter 9

Vincent Frank Bedogne, *Evolution of Consciousness*

Allan Coombs, *The Radiance of Being*

Riane Eisler, *The Chalice and the Blade*

Jean Gebser, *The Ever-Present Origin*

Gary Lachman, *A Secret History of Consciousness*

Steven Pinker, *The Better Angels of our Nature*

Paul Ray and Sherry Anderson, *The Cultural Creatives*
Pierre Teilhard de Chardin, *The Phenomenon of Man*

APPENDIX B

Universal Human Needs and Feelings/Emotions lists. Reprinted with credit to and permission from baynvc.org.

UNIVERSAL HUMAN NEEDS

SUBSISTENCE AND SECURITY

Physical Sustenance
Air
Food
Health
Movement
Physical Safety
Rest/Sleep
Shelter
Touch
Water

Security
Consistency
Order/Structure
Peace (external)
Peace of mind
Protection
Safety (emotional)
Stability
Trusting

FREEDOM
Autonomy
Choice
Ease
Independence
Power
Self-responsibility
Space
Spontaneity

Leisure/Relaxation
Humor
Joy
Play
Pleasure
Rejuvenation

Connection
Affection
Appreciation
Attention
Closeness

Companionship
Harmony
Intimacy
Love
Nurturing
Sexual Expression
Support
Tenderness
Warmth

To Matter
Acceptance
Care
Compassion
Consideration
Empathy
Kindness
Mutual Recognition
Respect
  To be heard, to be
  seen, to be
  known, to be un-

derstood,
to be trusted
Understanding
others

Community
Belonging
Communication
Cooperation
Equality
Inclusion
Mutuality
Participation
Partnership
Self-expression
Sharing

MEANING
Sense of Self
Authenticity
Competence
Creativity

Dignity
Growth
Healing
Honesty
Integrity
Self-acceptance
Self-care
Self-connection
Self-knowledge
Self-realization
Matter to myself

Understanding
Awareness
Clarity
Discovery
Learning
Making sense of
life
Stimulation

Meaning

Aliveness
Challenge
Consciousness
Contribution
Creativity
Effectiveness
Exploration
Integration
Purpose

Transcendence
Beauty
Celebration of life
Communion
Faith
Flow
Hope
Inspiration
Mourning
Peace (internal)
Presence

This list builds on Marshall Rosenberg's original needs list with categories adapted from Manfred Max-Neef. Neither exhaustive nor definitive, it can be used for study and for discovery about each person's authentic experience. Composed in 2009 by Inbal, Miki, and Arnina Kashtan, baynvc.org, (510) 433-0700. For the fullest description of the way Miki Kashtan uses the concepts of feelings and needs, see her book *Spinning Threads of Radical Aliveness and Reweaving Our Human Fabric.*

FEELINGS/EMOTIONS—PARTIAL LIST

(internal sensations, without reference to
thoughts, interpretations)

*We use the following words when we want to express a combination
of mental states and physical sensations. This list is neither exhaustive
nor definitive. It is meant as a starting place to support anyone who
wishes to engage in a process of deepening self-discovery, and to facilitate greater understanding and connection between people.*

A. FEELINGS WE MAY EXPERIENCE WHEN OUR NEEDS ARE BEING MET:

AFFECTIONATE	ENGAGED	animated
compassionate	absorbed	ardent
friendly	alert	aroused
loving	curious	dazzled
openhearted	engrossed	eager
sympathetic	enchanted	energetic
tender	entranced	enthusiastic
warm	fascinated	giddy
	interested	invigorated
	intrigued	lively
CONFIDENT	involved	passionate
	spellbound	surprised
empowered	stimulated	vibrant
open		
proud		EXHILARATED
safe	EXCITED	blissful
secure	amazed	ecstatic

elated

enthralled

exuberant

radiant

rapturous

thrilled

GRATEFUL

appreciative

moved

thankful

touched

HOPEFUL

expectant

encouraged

optimistic

JOYFUL

amused

delighted

glad

happy

jubilant

pleased

tickled

INSPIRED

amazed

awed

wonder

PEACEFUL

calm

clearheaded

comfortable

centered

content

equanimity

fulfilled

mellow

quiet

relaxed

relieved

satisfied

serene

still

tranquil

trusting

REFRESHED

enlivened

rejuvenated

renewed

rested

restored

revived

B. FEELINGS WE MAY EXPERIENCE WHEN OUR NEEDS ARE *NOT* BEING MET:

AFRAID

apprehensive

dread

foreboding

frightened

mistrustful

panicked

petrified

scared

suspicious

terrified

wary

worried

ANNOYED

aggravated
dismayed
disgruntled
displeased
exasperated
frustrated
impatient
irritated
irked

ANGRY

angry
enraged
furious
incensed
indignant
irate
livid
outraged
resentful

AVERSION

animosity
appalled
contempt
disgusted
dislike
hate

horrified
hostile
repulsed

CONFUSED

ambivalent
baffled
bewildered
dazed
hesitant
lost
mystified
perplexed
puzzled
torn

DISCONNECTED

alienated
aloof
apathetic
bored
cold
detached
distant
distracted
indifferent
numb
removed

withdrawn

DISQUIET

agitated
alarmed
discombobulated
disconcerted
disturbed
perturbed
rattled
restless
shocked
startled
surprised
troubled
turbulent
turmoil
uncomfortable
uneasy
unnerved
unsettled
upset

EMBARRASSED

ashamed
chagrined
flustered
mortified

self-conscious

FATIGUE

beat

burnt out

depleted

exhausted

lethargic

listless

sleepy

tired

weary

worn out

PAIN

agony

anguished

bereaved

devastated

grief

heartbroken

hurt

lonely

miserable

regretful

remorseful

SAD

depressed

dejected

despair

despondent

disappointed

discouraged

disheartened

forlorn

gloomy

heavy hearted

hopeless

melancholy

unhappy

wretched

TENSE

anxious

cranky

distressed

distraught

edgy

fidgety

frazzled

irritable

jittery

nervous

overwhelmed

restless

stressed out

VULNERABLE

fragile

guarded

helpless

insecure

leery

reserved

sensitive

shaky

YEARNING

envious

jealous

longing

nostalgic

pining

wistful

This list is a collaborative effort of many, and adapted from Marshall Rosenberg's original list. Copyright © 2008 by Inbal Kashtan and Miki Kashtan.

www.ingramcontent.com/pod-product-compliance
Lightning Source LLC
Chambersburg PA
CBHW021618270326
41931CB00008B/751